DIETITIANS OF CANADA
GREAT FOOD FAST

Bev Callaghan, RD • Lynn Roblin, RD

DIETITIANS OF CANADA
GREAT FOOD FAST

Bev Callaghan, RD • Lynn Roblin, RD

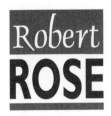

Robert
ROSE

Great Food Fast

DESIGN, EDITORIAL AND PRODUCTION:	MATTHEWS COMMUNICATIONS DESIGN INC.
PHOTOGRAPHY:	MARK T. SHAPIRO
ART DIRECTION, FOOD PHOTOGRAPHY:	SHARON MATTHEWS
FOOD STYLIST:	KATE BUSH
PROP STYLIST:	CHARLENE ERRICSON
MANAGING EDITOR:	PETER MATTHEWS
INDEX:	BARBARA SCHON
COLOR SCANS & FILM:	POINTONE GRAPHICS

Cover photo: SKILLET CHICKEN AND SHRIMP PAELLA (PAGE 132)

We acknowledge the financial support of the Government of Canada through the Book Publishing Industry Development Program (BPIDP) for our publishing activities. Canadä

Canadian Cataloguing in Publication Data

Callaghan, Bev
 Great food fast

Includes index.
ISBN 0-7788-0018-0

1. Quick and easy cookery. I. Roblin, Lynn. II. Dietitians of Canada. III. Title.

TX833.5.C34 2000	641.5'55	C00-930063-5

Published by: Robert Rose Inc. • 156 Duncan Mill Road, Suite 12
Toronto, Ontario, Canada M3B 2N2 Tel: (416) 449-3535

Printed in Canada
 234567 BP 03 02 01 00

CONTENTS

THANKS TO OUR SPONSORS

Dietitians of Canada gratefully acknowledges the three official sponsors and the media sponsor for their support of this cookbook and the Year 2000 National Nutrition Month campaign. The involvement of the Canadian Egg Marketing Agency, Dairy Farmers of Canada, Post Cereals and Chatelaine has been instrumental in making *Great Food Fast* a reality. All of these companies have a commitment to healthy eating messages that benefit all Canadians.

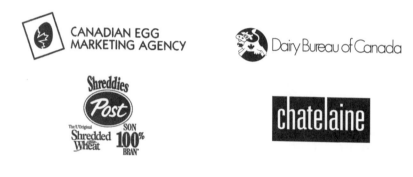

ABOUT DIETITIANS OF CANADA

Dietitians of Canada (DC) is the national voice of dietitians, working to improve the health of Canadians through food and nutrition. Representing more than 5,000 dietitians across Canada, DC is the third-largest national dietetic association in the world.

Dietitians are the ideal source of up-to-date, reliable nutrition advice. If you need healthy eating information or personal advice about your diet, contact a Registered Dietitian.

To find a Registered Dietitian in your community, contact your local department of public health, community health center, or hospital. You can also get a list of Registered Dietitians who work in private practice on the Dietitians of Canada website *www.dietitians.ca* or by calling the Consulting Dietitians Network at 1-888-901-7776.

 Dietitians of Canada
Les diététistes du Canada

Introduction

Welcome to *Great Food Fast* – the third cookbook from Dietitians of Canada. As the title says, this book focuses on preparing food that's quick and easy, healthy and delicious. The recipes are tried-and-true favorites from kitchens across the country. Try them and you'll discover that good nutrition doesn't require a lot of fuss. And it tastes great!

These days, time is an increasingly precious resource. And whether you are single, a couple or part of a family, the demands of work and personal life often leave little time for planning and preparing healthy meals.

Sure, you know that good nutrition is important. But so is convenience. Well, now you don't have to choose one or the other. In this book you'll find quick and easy meal solutions to get you through the day and encourage good eating habits for your family that will last a lifetime.

According to a recent study (*Speaking of Food and Eating Report: A Consumer Perspective,* Canadian Foundation for Dietetic Research, Dietitians of Canada and Kraft Canada Inc.), 60% of primary meal preparers agree that trying to decide what to cook is the worst part of meal preparation. And what are the most important factors in making that decision? For 68% it is ease of preparation; for 66% it's preparation time.

The study also found that a majority (56%) of Canadians are tired of getting conflicting messages about healthy eating.

And it *is* confusing. But that's where dietitians can help. So we've assembled this collection of recipes and proven nutrition tips to help you meet the challenge of preparing nutritious meals.

Enjoy great-tasting, nutritious food – fast!

Lise Smedmor, RD
National Nutrition Month Coordinator
Dietitians of Canada

Acknowledgements

Dietitians of Canada would like to thank the many people who have helped to produce this cookbook. First, a big thank you to all the people across Canada who submitted their recipes for our consideration. The response was overwhelming and the diversity and range of recipes were wonderful.

Next, of course, are our authors: Lynn Roblin, RD, MSc, who wrote the nutrition content, and Bev Callaghan, RD, who tested and developed the recipes. Our thanks also to Barbara Selley, RD and Sharyn Joliat, RD, MSc., of Info Access Inc. (1988) for the nutrient analysis. Bev and Lynn are grateful to Margie Armstrong, Mary Persi and Marilena Rutka for their expert assistance with all of the recipe testing and development; to Barbara McHughan for her help typing the cookbook manuscript; and to Meredith Jackson, RD, for reviewing the content. They would also like to thank their families, especially their children, for their patience and support.

We are deeply indebted to the DC members who reviewed the book for nutrition content and accuracy:

Zita Bersenas-Cers, RD, Hamilton, ON;

Bonnie Conrad, P.Dt. M.A.HE., Halifax, NS;

Renée Crompton, RD MSc., Ottawa, ON;

Janice Holley, RD, Morriston, ON;

Valerie Irvine, P.Dt., Saskatoon, SK;

Anar Jamal, RD, Calgary, AB;

Susan Mah, RD MHSc., Toronto, ON;

Mary Fodor O'Brien, RD MHSc., Oakville, ON;

Elizabeth Thomas, RDN, Abbotsford, BC;

Mary Sue Waisman, RD MSc., Calgary, AB;

Leslie Whittington-Carter, RD, London, ON.

Thank you to the dietitians and staff of the National Nutrition Month Campaign sponsors for their input: Anne Kennedy, RD, MHSc., Nutrition Manager, Canadian Egg Marketing Agency; Gail Ewan, P.Dt, MSc. and Susan Iantorno, RD, MHSc., Dairy Farmers of Canada; Marilynn Small, RD, Senior Nutrition Manager, Nutrition Affairs Kraft Canada Inc.; and Lindsey Davis, Assistant Brand Manager, Post Cereals.

A special thank you to Helen Haresign, RD, MSc., Director Development, Dietitians of Canada, for her guidance and leadership throughout the process of creating this cookbook. Thanks also to Lise Smedmor, RD, of L.M.C. Communications for coordinating the often complex tasks involved.

Finally, our thanks to publisher Robert Rose Inc., particularly Bob Dees; to Matthews Communications Design Inc. for their editorial, design and production expertise; to photographer Mark Shapiro, for his skill in making the food images look great; to Kate Bush for her formidable food-styling; and to Charlene Erricson, for finding the props that appear in the food photographs.

Getting Great Food Fast

Most of us care about what we eat and try to make the best possible food choices for our health. But hectic schedules often force us to skip meals, eat on the run, or quickly throw together a meal using foods close at hand. Some "grab-and-go" foods are fine – a piece of fruit, for example, or a bowl of cereal, some yogurt, or a sandwich. But as often as not we turn to high-fat snacks, fast foods, or prepared dishes to get a meal quickly. The result? We may not get the nutrients we need.

So don't let time constraints keep you from enjoying healthy eating. Here you'll find plenty of ideas to help you get great taste and nutrition – all in less time than you ever imagined possible.

What makes great food *great*?

Let's start with what it's not. A great meal doesn't have to be complicated. It doesn't have to be a hot meal and need not adhere to the old-fashioned "meat and two vegetables" concept. A balanced breakfast, even if eaten on the run, can still be great food. So can a quick energizing snack – or a more substantial meal eaten with friends or family.

Basically, a great meal is one that's nutritionally balanced and tastes delicious. Both qualities are important but, seeing as we're dietitians, let's consider nutrition first.

Great nutrition. Here, balance is the key. And in this book you'll find recipes that provide a wide range of essential nutrients. In fact, each recipe has been analyzed to provide you with information about the calories, protein, fat, carbohydrate, fiber and sodium content of each meal. Excellent and good sources of vitamins and minerals are also indicated. Balance also means eating foods from a variety of food groups. So each recipe lists the number of servings it contains of each food group as outlined in *Canada's Food Guide to Healthy Eating* (see page 176).

Great taste. The recipes in this book have been specially selected to provide a variety of cooking styles, flavors and textures – ranging from familiar favorites to dishes that are a little more unusual. Try them all, because they're all delicious. Be adventurous, get out of a rut and try something new. It can be a new ingredient, a new recipe or a new method of cooking.

Budget-friendly. Great food is even better when it doesn't cost a fortune. And here you'll find recipes that use everyday, mostly inexpensive ingredients available at your local supermarket.

What makes great food *fast?*

Surveys have shown that more and more people want nutritious, home-cooked meals – and they want them fast. So we've selected recipes for this book that can be prepared in a hurry. In fact, while cooking times vary with the type of meal, most recipes require only 10 to 30 minutes of preparation time.

Keep it short. For most recipes, ingredient lists have been kept as short as possible.

Keep it simple. Cooking instructions are easy to follow – easy enough that older children, teens and beginner cooks can help with meal preparation.

Take a few shortcuts. Commercially prepared ingredients, such as frozen vegetables or bottled pasta sauce, are sometimes used to save time in the kitchen.

VARIETY
the secret to eating well

It's normal to eat when we are hungry, eat quickly and eat the same foods over and over again. To save time, many of us rely on the same 5 to 10 main weekday meals.

Increasing the variety of foods you eat can improve your overall nutritional health. For example, when you eat a greater variety of whole grains, fruit and vegetables, you'll enjoy many different vitamins, minerals and fiber.

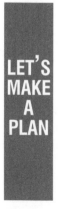

LET'S MAKE A PLAN

A weekly meal plan can help you get organized, cut down on trips to the store, and reduce reliance on take-out or delivered foods. If meal planning is a chore for you, at least think about the kinds of meals you would like to have over the next few days and make sure you have the ingredients on hand to make them.

Consider your weekly schedule

❧ **Breakfast and lunch meals** may need to be eaten quickly, on the run or taken in a lunch bag. For those occasions you'll need to stock up on simple portable foods. Check out the recipes and tips in "Getting off to a Great Start" (pages 27 to 44) and "Quick Meals and Snacks" (pages 45 to 64). Most of these recipes are simple enough for teens to make, serve and enjoy with their friends.

❧ **Weekday meals** have to be fast and easy. Making parts of meals ahead of time (see PIQUANT TOMATO SAUCE, page 150), using some convenience foods (see FAST CHILI, page 106), or planning to incorporate leftovers (see EGG AND MUSHROOM FRIED RICE, page 54) can help make weekday meal preparation easier. For ideas check out the recipes in "Super Soups" (pages 65 to 76), "Salads and Vegetables" (pages 77 to 99) and "Main Meals" (pages 100 to 154).

❧ **By the time Friday rolls around,** many of us are ready to take a break and order foods in. There's nothing wrong with this once in a while. We all need an occasional break from cooking.

❧ **On the weekend** there's often more time to cook and enjoy meals with family and friends. There might also be time to get a head start on busy weekday meals by making some meals ahead or making double batches of some recipes and freezing them for another day (LAZY LASAGNA, page 108, for example, or CARIBBEAN HAM AND BLACK BEAN SOUP, page 70). There are some great recipes for family meals and entertaining in "Main Meals" (pages 100 to 154). You'll also find some delicious dessert ideas in "Fast Finishes" (pages 155 to 171).

Check out the Sample Meal Plans (pages 172 to 173) for ideas on how to combine recipes from this book.

Planning points

- Build meals that include foods from each of the four food groups as outlined in *Canada's Food Guide to Healthy Eating* (see pages 176 to 177) or plan meals using the recipes in this book.

- Look for meals with plenty of grains, vegetables and fruit – these foods should make up about two-thirds of every meal.

- Use the "Great Food Fast Pantry List" (at right) as a guide for stocking up on basic ingredients and healthy food choices.

- Make a shopping list and add items that you will need for breakfasts, lunches and snacks. Keep a running list on the fridge to add items you need or use up.

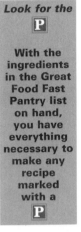

Look for the

P

With the ingredients in the Great Food Fast Pantry list on hand, you have everything necessary to make any recipe marked with a

P

- Decide on three or four main meals you can make during the week. Add to your shopping list any food items you need to make these meals.

- Be flexible about your meal plans so that you or your helpers have a choice about what to make for dinner. Keep in mind that some foods (such as dairy products, fresh fish, poultry and meat) are more perishable than others and will need to be used up first.

- Post your meal plan on the refrigerator so that whoever gets home first can start the meal. Have your cookbook opened to the right recipe page so directions are readily accessible.

- On days when you know you won't have time to cook, plan to serve leftovers or meals that can be made ahead of time.

KEEP A WELL-STOCKED PANTRY

Having a good supply of simple, nutritious foods in your cupboards, fridge and freezer ensures that you'll have everything you need to make meals in a hurry. The following includes some of the key ingredients used to make the recipes in this book. Stock up on these pantry items to get a head start on your meal-making.

PANTRY LIST

In the cupboard ...

Beans and lentils, canned: baked beans in tomato sauce, black beans, kidney beans, chickpeas, white pea or navy beans, lentils

Bread: whole grain breads, rolls, pita bread, bagels, biscuit baking mix

Cereals: bran, whole grain, quick rolled oats

Condiments and flavorings: mustard, ketchup, vinegar, soya sauce, bouillon cubes

Fish, canned: tuna, salmon, clams

Flour: white and whole grain

Fruit, canned (packed in juice or light syrup): peaches, pears, pineapple, mandarin orange segments, applesauce

Fruit, dried: raisins, cranberries, apricots, dates

Herbs and spices: pepper, basil, garlic, ginger, oregano, thyme, tarragon, coriander and cumin

Milk, canned evaporated, skim powdered

Nuts and seeds: almonds, walnuts, peanuts

Oil: olive oil, vegetable oil

Pasta: fusilli, rotini, spaghetti, penne, bow-ties, couscous

Pasta sauces: prepared tomato and vegetable

Rice: white or brown, quick-cooking rice

Sweeteners: sugar, honey, syrup, jam

Vegetables, canned: stewed or diced tomatoes, corn kernels, pumpkin

Vegetables, fresh: potatoes, sweet potatoes, onions

Vegetables, pickled: sweet pickles, dill pickles

Wheat bran, cornmeal

continued next page...

PANTRY LIST

On the counter ...

Bananas, cantaloupe, tomatoes

In the fridge ...

Cheese: Cheddar, Parmesan, ricotta, mozzarella, cheese slices

Eggs

Fats: margarine, butter

Fruit, fresh: oranges, kiwi, apples, grapes, pears

Juice: tomato, vegetable, fruit, lemon

Meat and poultry: chicken, turkey, beef, lean ground beef, pork chops (freeze poultry and meat if you can't use within two days of purchasing)

Milk: skim, 1%, 2%, whole milk, or buttermilk

Vegetables: carrots, red and green bell peppers, broccoli, romaine lettuce, celery, spinach, green onions, mushrooms, zucchini

Yogurt: plain and flavored

In the freezer ...

Bread: pita bread, flour tortillas, flat bread rounds

Frozen fish and seafood: sole, perch, halibut, haddock, cooked shrimp

Fruit: strawberries, raspberries, blueberries

Fruit juice concentrate

Vegetables, plain or mixed: peas, corn, broccoli and cauliflower, oriental mix

Personalize this list by adding the ingredients for your favorite recipes.

❧ For best flavor (and price!), purchase fresh fruit and vegetables in season; if possible, choose locally grown produce.

❧ Buy only what you can use or preserve in the next few days; once fresh produce starts to wilt or spoil, it loses nutrients and flavor.

❧ Consider frozen vegetables as a convenient and economical alternative to fresh; they are just as nutritious, keep well and reduce chopping and preparation time. Go easy on frozen vegetables packed in sauce; they tend to be higher in fat.

❧ Canned vegetables are useful to have on hand; they usually contain added salt, however, so check the label if you need to watch your sodium intake.

❧ When fresh fruit is not available (or too expensive) buy frozen fruit or canned fruit packed in juice or light syrup. Try unsweetened applesauce as a substitute for fresh apples.

❧ Instead of fruit drinks, cocktails or punches, choose real fruit juices – reconstituted or frozen concentrate; they contain more nutrients.

Shopping tips

When buying grain products:

❧ Select breads and cereals made from whole wheat, bran, oats, rye, or mixed grains. They contain more fiber than those made with white flour. Check labels to compare fiber content (see "What Nutrition Claims Really Mean," page 13).

❧ Choose croissants, doughnuts, pastries and cookies less often. These often contain a lot of extra fat.

❧ Try to limit flavored rice and pasta mixes; they may be higher in sodium.

When buying vegetables and fruit:

❧ Choose a variety of red, orange or dark green vegetables and fruit; they usually contain more nutrients than those with lighter colors.

When buying milk products:

❧ Check labels for percent butterfat (% B.F.) or milk fat (% M.F.); the lower the number, the less fat you get.

❧ Different types of plain and flavored yogurt can vary considerably in fat content. Those with 2% M.F. or less are lower in fat.

❧ Buy regular or lower-fat cheeses such as Cheddar, mozzarella, brick and colby.

❧ Choose yogurt or use light sour cream, which contains half the fat (or less) found in the regular product.

❧ Use cream cheese in moderation; it is higher in fat and provides little or no calcium.

When buying meat and alternatives:

❧ Select lean varieties such as skinless chicken, turkey breast, pork tenderloin or chops, flank steaks, beef round roasts, lean or extra lean ground beef; also, choose lean deli meats such as turkey breast, chicken, roast beef, ham and pastrami.

❧ Choose from a variety of fresh or frozen fish – such as sole, perch, haddock, halibut or salmon – as well as shrimp and canned salmon or tuna packed in water.

❧ Look for eggs classified as Canada Grade "A" – and make sure they have been properly refrigerated.

❧ Buy canned or dried beans, peas and lentils; they are an inexpensive source of protein, low in fat and high in fiber.

❧ Include some nuts and seeds such as almonds, pecans, peanuts, sesame seeds and nut butters – that is, unless someone in the household has nut allergies.

Understanding food labels

Food labels provide three important types of information that can help you make good choices.

Nutrition claims. These are statements about the key benefits of a food product. Examples include "low in fat" or "fat-free" or "high in fiber" or "a source of 7 essential nutrients." These claims must meet strict criteria and, when used, must be supported by detailed nutrition information on the label. (See "What Nutrition Claims Really Mean," at right.) The nutrition-claims criteria have been used to provide nutrition information about the recipes in this book. For example, CHUNKY VEGETABLE LENTIL SOUP (see recipe, page 73) is considered "low in fat" and "high in fiber."

Nutrition information panel. Here you'll find quantitative nutrition information, including the number of calories, as well as the amount of pro-

tein, fat, carbohydrates and other nutrients for a given serving of the food.

Ingredient list. This shows the ingredients of the food product, listed in descending order of amount (weight) used. The ingredient list can help you compare products or choose more nutrient-rich foods. For example, a loaf of bread that lists whole wheat flour as the first ingredient will be higher in fiber than one that lists white flour first. Ingredient lists can also help you identify substances to which you or members of your family may be allergic.

WHAT NUTRITION CLAIMS really mean

- **"Low in fat"** or **"Low-fat."** Contains no more than 3 g fat per serving.
- **"Fat-free."** Contains no more that 0.5 g fat per serving.
- **"Moderate source of fiber"** or **"A source of fiber."** Contains at least 2 g dietary fiber per serving.
- **"High in fiber."** Contains at least 4 g dietary fiber per serving.
- **"Very high in fiber."** Contains at least 6 g dietary fiber per serving.
- **"Salt-free"** or **"Sodium-free."** Contains less than or equal to 5 mg sodium/100 g of food.
- **"Source of"** a vitamin or mineral. Contains at least 5% of the recommended daily intake of that vitamin or mineral per serving.
- **"Good source of"** or **"High in"** a vitamin or mineral. Contains at least 15% of the recommended daily intake of that vitamin or mineral or, in the case of vitamin C, 30% of the recommended daily intake per serving.
- **"Excellent source of"** or **"Very high in"** a vitamin or mineral. Contains at least 25% of the recommended daily intake of that vitamin or mineral or, in the case of vitamin C, 50% of the recommended daily intake per serving.

Source: **Guide to Food Labelling and Advertising.** Canadian Food Inspection Agency, March 1996.

Watch the serving size.

A product may be "low in fat" per serving but if you eat a number of servings, those grams of fat can really add up!

Fat-free does not mean calorie-free.

Just because a food is "fat-free" don't be fooled into thinking you can eat as much as you like. Many of these foods contain a significant number of calories.

Safety first

All too often, people suffer from food-related illnesses caused by poor food handling, not cooking food to the correct temperature, or eating food that has been contaminated with bacteria.

Here's how to make sure your food is safe to eat:

- Wash hands, utensils and surfaces with hot soapy water before, during and after food preparation. Remember, too, that wet hands can transmit bacteria, so be sure to dry them thoroughly.

- Always sanitize countertops, cutting boards and utensils with a mild bleach and water solution (one capful of bleach per sink full of clean rinse water), especially after preparing raw meat, fish, poultry or eggs.

- To avoid contamination, keep raw meat, fish and poultry drippings away from other foods during preparation and refrigeration.

- Store, serve and reheat foods at safe temperatures: below 4° C (40° F) for cold foods and above 60° C (140° F) for hot foods. Discard all foods that have been sitting at room temperature for over 2 hours. Leftovers should be refrigerated immediately in shallow containers to ensure rapid cooling.

- Use packaged foods prior to the "best before" date. (Remember that, once opened, a food's "best before" date no longer applies.) Use fresh foods as quickly as possible. If cheese is mouldy or eggs are cracked, discard them. Refrigerated leftovers generally should be used within 3 days. For more information, see "How Long Will it Keep?" (page 174).

- Defrost meat, poultry and seafood in the refrigerator or microwave – not on the counter where, as the outer surfaces of the food warm up, bacteria multiply quickly. If you thaw meat in the microwave, cook it immediately.

- Cook meats, poultry and fish thoroughly and put them on a clean plate – not on the one that held these foods before they were cooked.

- When in doubt – throw it out!

For more information on food safety, check out the Canadian Partnership for Food Safety Education website at *www.canfightbac.org.*

Getting Great Nutrition

E ating well is one of the cornerstones of a healthy lifestyle. Good nutrition contributes to normal growth and development and keeps you feeling and looking your best.

When you combine good nutrition with other healthy lifestyle habits – such as keeping active and reducing stress (the two often go hand in hand), not smoking and using alcohol in moderation – you have the best chance of protecting your long-term health.

But getting great nutrition goes beyond eating simply for energy and nutrients. It's not only what you eat, but how you eat. Eating well means taking the time to enjoy foods and share mealtimes with friends or family whenever possible.

Look good, feel great

The elements of good nutrition are the same for anyone in generally good health, and they're found in *Canada's Guidelines for Healthy Eating**. Follow these simple rules for healthy eating to look and feel great, avoid being overweight and help prevent future health problems such as heart disease, cancer and osteoporosis.

The *Guidelines** say:
- Enjoy a variety of foods.
- Emphasize cereals, breads, other grain products, vegetables and fruit.
- Choose lower-fat dairy products, leaner meats and foods prepared with little or no fat.
- Achieve and maintain a healthy body weight by enjoying regular physical activity and healthy eating.
- Limit salt, alcohol and caffeine.

* *Source: Health and Welfare Canada, 1990*

GETTING THE GOODS
Key nutrients in the four food groups

Food Group	Key Nutrients
Grain Products	Carbohydrate, fiber, protein, thiamin, riboflavin, niacin, folacin, iron, zinc, magnesium
Vegetables & Fruit	Carbohydrate, fiber, thiamin, folacin, vitamin A, vitamin C, iron, magnesium
Milk Products	Protein, fat, riboflavin, vitamin B_{12}, vitamin A, vitamin D, calcium, zinc, magnesium
Meat & Alternatives	Protein, fat, thiamin, riboflavin, niacin, folacin, vitamin B_{12}, iron, zinc, magnesium

Follow the Food Guide

For helpful advice on choosing what foods to eat (and how much), check out *Canada's Food Guide to Healthy Eating*. This guide (reproduced in full on page 176) is based on selecting foods from the four food groups – Grain Products, Vegetables & Fruit, Milk Products, and Meat & Alternatives. Each group provides a unique set of essential nutrients (see chart, page 15). That's why it's important to choose foods from all these groups each day, as well as a variety of foods within each group.

The myth of "bad" foods

No single food should be considered bad or harmful to health. Healthy eating habits are not made or destroyed by one food, meal, or day's worth of eating. What matters most to your health is what you eat regularly from day to day. If you haven't eaten as well as you should, just make healthier choices for your following meals and snacks. Just remember, all foods can be part of healthy eating. Moderation is the key.

Foods," and include things like fats and oils, margarine and butter, potato or corn chips (and other high-fat and/or high-salt snack foods), sugar, jam, syrup, candy, chocolate and other sweets, water, coffee, tea, soft drinks, alcohol, herbs, spices and condiments.

Does this mean you shouldn't eat these foods? Certainly not. While not as essential to nutrition, these foods can add to the taste and enjoyment of meals and snacks, and are often eaten with foods from one or more of the four food groups. Many are higher in fat or calories, however, so use them in moderation.

Balance is one of the most important elements of good nutrition. A balanced meal is one that includes something from each of the four food groups.

To help you provide balanced meals, each recipe in this book features a chart that shows the number of Food Guide servings in that recipe.

In some cases a meal may only include three out of the four food groups. That is because you may be able to satisfy your daily requirements at other meals or snacks.

Also, you'll find that most recipes give suggestions to "Complete the Meal" – in other words, to add foods that ensure all four food groups are included.

Outside the Group

Take a look at *Canada's Food Guide to Healthy Eating* (see page 176) and you'll notice that there are many foods and beverages that don't belong to any food group. These are classified as "Other

Questions of quantity

Eating the right amount of food helps you satisfy your nutrient needs and maintain a healthy weight. But how much food do you need? The answer depends on your age, gender and activity level, and whether you are pregnant or breastfeeding.

Canada's Food Guide to Healthy Eating (see page 176) provides general guidelines for how much food to eat and specifies a range of recommended servings and typical serving sizes. Here's how it can work for different people:

Young children and **older women who are not very active** should aim for the lower number of servings from each food group each day (for example, 5 servings of Grain Products, 5 servings of Vegetables & Fruit, 2 servings of Milk Products and 2 servings of Meat & Alternatives). Children under the age of four can be given the same number of servings, but smaller serving sizes. A typical serving for a preschooler is about half of a regular serving.

Moderately active women and **sedentary men** can choose somewhere towards the middle of the range for each food group (for example, 6 servings of Grain Products, 7 servings of Vegetables & Fruit, 2 to 4 servings of Milk Products and 2 to 3 servings of Meat & Alternatives).

Very active males and females will probably require the higher number of servings in the recommended range (for example, 12 servings of Grain Products, 10 servings of Vegetables & Fruit, 4 servings of Milk Products and 3 servings of Meat & Alternatives).

Family feeding

Whenever possible, enjoy your meals with family and friends. This is an important part of healthy eating because people who eat together generally eat more balanced meals and a greater variety of foods. There is also time to talk and – better still! – you'll be able to share the work of preparing meals and cleaning up.

For parents concerned about their children's nutrition, it's important to remember that taste preferences and eating habits start to form early in life and are strongly influenced by family and peers. Children's nutrient intakes often mirror their parents', so it's important for parents to serve as good role models for healthy eating and to make healthy choices available.

the Essentials of Great Nutrition

The key nutrients of healthy eating are carbohydrate, protein, fat, vitamins and minerals. These essential nutrients help your body grow, function properly and stay healthy. Fiber and water, although not nutrients as such, are also important.

Carbohydrates

Carbohydrates are the principal source of energy for your body and should account for over half of your daily food choices.

Complex carbohydrate foods are among the most important because they provide you with important vitamins, minerals, fiber and other substances. Complex carbohydrate foods include whole grain breads and cereals, rice, pasta, some vegetables, (potatoes, corn, and peas) and dried beans, peas and lentils.

Eating patterns that are high in complex carbohydrates and fiber have been shown to help in the prevention of many diseases such as heart disease and some types of cancer.

Simple carbohydrate foods include those that are nutrient-rich (milk, fruit, vegetables), and "Other Foods" such as sugar, honey, jam, candies, fruit-flavored beverages and soft drinks. These "Other Foods" can be part of a healthy diet but shouldn't replace more nutritious choices.

Focus on **Fiber**

Dietary fiber is found only in plant foods. It can help maintain a healthy digestive system and aid in controlling blood cholesterol, blood sugar and weight. Two types of fiber are important to our health: *insoluble fiber* helps promote bowel function; *soluble fiber* plays a role in lowering blood cholesterol levels and controlling blood sugar levels in people with diabetes. Foods containing these different types of fiber are shown below:

Type of fiber	Food examples
Insoluble fiber	wheat bran, whole grain products and some vegetables
Soluble fiber	grains such as oats, barley, psyllium; dried beans, peas and lentils; some vegetables and fruit

Most Canadians don't consume enough fiber. Adults should aim for 25 to 35 g of fiber per day. For children aged 3 to 18, daily recommended fiber intake (in grams) can be calculated as the sum of their age plus 5. So, a 10 year old child, for example, should have $10 + 5 = 15$ grams of fiber per day.

Getting more fiber

As a general rule, try to make whole grains, vegetables and fruit part of every meal.

Choose breads and cereals containing wheat bran, whole wheat, oats, rye, flaxseeds, or mixed grains and brown rice. Use whole grain bagels, pita bread and flour tortilla wraps. And in recipes calling for white flour, try substituting up to half the amount with whole wheat flour.

Fruits and vegetables are a good source of fiber – even better if you keep skins on.

Other good sources of fiber include bean-based soups and salads, as well as main meals made with beans, peas, or lentils.

When using this book, look at the amount of fiber you get in each recipe and check to see how the different ingredients affect the fiber content. And when you're buying prepared foods, check labels and choose products with more grams of fiber per serving.

Health note: As you increase your fiber intake, be sure to drink more fluids (like water) to help the fiber work properly.

Fiber-full recipes

Here's a list of recipes in this book that are rated "very high in" dietary fiber.

Big-Batch Bran Muffins (page 33)

Creamy Microwave Oatmeal (page 37)

Breakfast Muesli to Go (page 39)

Lunch Box Chili Rice and Beans (page 55)

Lunch Box Peachy Sweet Potato and Couscous (page 56)

Beef, Vegetable and Bean Soup (page 69)

Tomato and Bean Soup (page 76)

Chicken and Bean Salad (page 81)

Triple-Bean, Rice and Artichoke Salad (page 93)

Fast Chili (page 106)

Chinese Almond Chicken with Noodles (page 124)

Spaghettini with Tuna, Olives and Capers (page 143)

Chickpea Hot Pot (page 145)

Crowd-Pleasing Vegetarian Chili (page 147)

Pasta with Roasted Vegetables and Goat Cheese (page 149)

Penne with Mushrooms and Spicy Tomato Sauce (page 151)

Rotini with Vegetable Tomato Sauce (page 152)

Country Apple Berry Crisp (page 162)

Protein

Protein is necessary for the growth, maintenance and repair of body tissues and for optimal health. Protein is something that isn't lacking in the typical North American diet. In fact, most people eat more than enough protein.

Protein is found primarily in animal products like milk products, meat, poultry, fish and eggs. Protein is also found in some plant products such as soy products, nuts, peanut butter, seeds, beans, peas and lentils.

Fat

While fat has developed a bad reputation in recent years, the fact is that some fat is necessary to maintain good health. The problem is when we eat too much fat, which can contribute to health problems.

Some fat facts:

❧ Fat provides energy (calories) and essential fatty acids and helps us absorb the fat-soluble vitamins A, D, E and K.

❧ Fat adds flavor and texture to many foods, making them more appealing to eat.

❧ Diets that are high in fat are often high in calories. Over the long term this can lead to weight gain and obesity, which increases the risk for heart disease, high blood pressure and diabetes.

❧ The suggested daily fat intake for women is 65 grams or less; for men it is 90 grams or less. (Figures are based on keeping fat intakes to less than 30% of calories.)

❧ Most Canadians still eat too much fat. To help reduce fat intake, look for lower-fat dairy products, leaner meats and foods prepared with little or no fat.

❧ Children need more fat in their diets than adults. Fat requirements decrease gradually from about 50% of calories from fat in infancy to about 30% of calories from fat in late adolescence. The extra fat children need should come from milk products, peanut butter, eggs and meat.

❧ Nutritious food for children should not be restricted because of fat content. Foods that provide extra fat and calories without the benefit of additional nutrients – such as deep-fried foods, chocolate bars, chips and other snack foods – should be used in moderation.

Types of fat

All fats are not the same. Here's a rundown on the different types of fat:

Saturated fat. Typically hard or solid at room temperature, this type of fat is found mostly in animal foods (meat, dairy products and lard), tropical oils (palm and coconut oil) and hydrogenated products (some margarine, cookies, crackers). High intakes of saturated fat tend to increase blood cholesterol levels, which is a risk factor for heart disease.

Trans-fatty acids. These occur naturally in some foods, but are also created when liquid fats are hardened by a process called *hydrogenation*. Like saturated fat, trans-fatty acids are thought to raise blood cholesterol. Foods containing partially hydrogenated vegetable oil include shortening, some margarines, some crackers, chips, cookies, bakery products, deep-fried chicken and fish, doughnuts and French fries.

Polyunsaturated fat. This type of fat is liquid even when refrigerated. It is found mostly in nuts and seeds, and in oils made from corn, safflower and sunflower, soybeans, nuts and seeds. It is also found in non-hydrogenated margarines.

Polyunsaturated fat has the beneficial effect of lowering blood cholesterol levels when eaten as part of a lower-fat diet.

Omega-3 fats are a type of polyunsaturated fat found in fish oils, some fish (salmon, sardines, tuna, herring, mackerel), flaxseeds and omega-3 enriched eggs. Omega-3 fatty acids tend to lower triglyceride levels.

Monounsaturated fat. Partially cloudy or partly solid if refrigerated, this type of fat is found mostly in canola, peanut and olive oils, in margarine made with these oils, as well as nut oils, nuts and seeds. It is thought to have a mild effect on lowering blood cholesterol

Cholesterol. Found in foods of animal origin, such as eggs, dairy products, meat and shellfish. At one time it was thought that high amounts of cholesterol from foods increased cholesterol levels in the blood. But now we know that a high intake of saturated fat has a much greater effect on increasing blood cholesterol levels than does cholesterol we eat.

Blood cholesterol is the cholesterol that circulates in your blood. Most of this cholesterol is produced in your liver. Dietary cholesterol comes from foods of animal origin. There is no cholesterol in plant foods.

Top 10 ways to cut down the fat

1. Make grains, vegetables and fruit the most substantial part of every meal.

2. Buy lower-fat milk products more often — buttermilk, skim, 1% milk or 2 % milk, or yogurt (2% M.F. or less) or cottage cheese (4% M.F. or less).

3. Try lower-fat cheeses such as part-skim mozzarella and light ricotta cheese or smaller amounts of strong-flavored cheeses (such as old Cheddar or Parmesan cheese).

4. Choose fish, poultry and lean meats; make sure excess fat is trimmed and/or skin is removed.

5. Use lower-fat cooking methods such as baking, broiling, roasting, grilling and microwaving.

6. Flavor foods with lemon, salsa, mustard, ketchup, herbs and spices.

7. Prepare foods without adding extra oil, butter, margarine, gravy or rich sauces.

8. Use poly- and monounsaturated oils more often than saturated fats.

9. Check recipes and product labels to see how much fat you get per serving.

10. Limit your servings of high-fat snack foods and rich desserts.

Vitamins

Vitamins promote normal growth and development, help release energy from food, fight infections, protect against damage to cells, and generally keep us healthy. (To see which foods supply these important nutrients, see the chart on page 15.)

Water-soluble vitamins. Vitamin C and the B-vitamins (thiamin, riboflavin, niacin, B_6, B_{12}, biotin, folacin and pantothenic acid) are water-soluble vitamins, which are not stored in your body for long periods. You need to get these vitamins from foods every day.

Fat-soluble vitamins. Vitamins A, D, E, and K are fat-soluble vitamins, which are stored in your body so it is less essential to get these in your diet each day.

Antioxidants. Vitamins C and E and beta-carotene (the plant form of vitamin A) are called antioxidant vitamins. These vitamins are thought to play an important role in protecting against heart disease and cancer.

Focus on Folic Acid

Folic acid (folacin) is a very important B vitamin that helps make new body cells and works with vitamin B_{12} to form hemoglobin in red blood cells. It also helps during pregnancy to prevent neural tube defects, such as spina bifida, in the fetus. (Women planning a pregnancy who have no history of neural tube defects should consider increasing their intake of folic acid through healthy food choices and a daily supplement containing 400 µg (0.4 mg) of folic acid.)

Food sources of folic acid*

Excellent sources include cooked beans, chickpeas, lentils, cooked spinach, asparagus, romaine lettuce, orange juice, canned pineapple juice, sunflower seeds.

Good sources include cooked lima beans, corn, bean sprouts, cooked broccoli, green peas, Brussels sprouts, beets, oranges, honeydew, raspberries, blackberries, avocado, roasted peanuts, wheat germ.

* Source: Health Canada, 1999

First in Folic Acid

Here's a list of recipes in this book rated "very high in" or "excellent source of" folic acid:

Sunny Orange Shake (page 30)

Overnight Broccoli and Cheese Strata (page 44)

Black Bean Salsa (page 48)

Lunch Box Chili Rice and Beans (page 55)

Lunch Box Peachy Sweet Potatoes and Couscous (page 56)

Swiss Chard Frittata in a Pita (page 62)

Beef, Vegetable and Bean Soup (page 69)

Caribbean Ham and Black Bean Soup (page 70)

Chunky Vegetable Lentil Soup (page 73)

Chicken and Bean Salad (page 81)

Colorful Bean and Corn Salad (page 83)

Fusilli and Fruit Salad (page 87)

Penne Salad with Asparagus and Tuna (page 90)

Triple Bean Salad with Rice and Artichokes (page 93)

Cauliflower Casserole (page 95)

Sautéed Spinach with Pine Nuts (page 99)

Fast Chili (page 106)

Lazy Lasagna page 108)

Pastitsio (page 110)

Veggie, Beef and Pasta Bake (page 114)

Creamy Bow-Tie Pasta with Chicken, Spinach and Peppers (page 126)

Hot 'n' Spicy Turkey Burgers (page 131)

Crunchy Fish Burgers (page 137)

Pasta with White Clam Sauce (page 139)

Quick Steamed Fish Fillets with Potatoes and Asparagus (page 140)

Salmon with Roasted Vegetables (page 141)

Shrimp and Mussels with Couscous (page 142)

Spaghettini with Tuna, Olives and Capers (page 143)

Chickpea Hot Pot (page 145)

Crowd-Pleasing Vegetarian Chili (page 147)

Fettuccine Carbonara (page 148)

Pasta with Roasted Vegetables and Goat Cheese (page 149)

Penne with Mushrooms and Spicy Tomato Sauce (page 151)

Rotini with Vegetable Tomato Sauce (page 152)

Spinach and Mushroom Pizza Pie (page 153)

Teriyaki Tofu Stir-Fry (page 154)

Minerals

Minerals help regulate fluid balance, muscle contractions and nerve impulses. They also play an important role in forming and maintaining healthy blood cells, bones and teeth. Like vitamins, minerals have their own unique functions. Important minerals include:

Calcium

This is important for healthy nerve function, blood clotting, muscle contraction, normal development and maintenance of strong bones and teeth. Calcium is important in helping to protect against osteoporosis, a condition in which bones become brittle and weak, most common in post-menopausal women. The best prevention is an adequate intake of calcium-rich foods and being active from an early age.

Milk and milk products are the most easily absorbed sources of calcium. *Canada's Food Guide to Healthy Eating* recommends 2 to 4 servings of milk products each day. Female teens and women should aim for the higher number of servings to help build calcium stores and protect themselves from osteoporosis. Individuals who don't consume milk products need to include plenty of other calcium-containing foods each day. However, these foods often contain much less calcium or calcium that is not absorbed well by the body.

Food sources of calcium*

Excellent source: firm cheeses, milk (fluid and dry), calcium fortified plant-based beverages, plain yogurt, canned sardines.

Good source: feta cheese, flavored yogurt, cheese slices, tofu set with calcium sulphate, almonds, canned salmon with bones.

Source: ricotta cheese, cooked or canned legumes, cooked oysters, sesame seeds, dried sunflower seeds, creamed cottage cheese, cooked bok choy, turnip greens.

Spinach, chard, beet greens, sweet potatoes and rhubarb are poor sources of calcium. These foods (as well as legumes and bran products) contain oxalate or phytate, which inhibit calcium absorption.

* *Source: Canada Nutrient File, Health Canada, 1997*

Cooking for Calcium

Here's a list of recipes in this book rated "very high in" or "excellent source of" calcium.

Sunny Orange Shake (page 30)

Banana-Berry Wake-Up Shake (page 31)

Creamy Microwave Oatmeal (page 37)

Breakfast Muesli to Go (page 39)

Overnight Broccoli and Cheese Strata (page 44)

Swiss Chard Frittata in a Pita (page 62)

Seafood Chowder (page 74)

Tomato and Bean Soup (page 76)

Cauliflower Casserole (page 95)

Lazy Lasagna (page 108)

Baked Chicken Parmesan (page 123)

Creamy Bow-Tie Pasta with Chicken, Spinach and Peppers (page 126)

Fettuccine Carbonara (page 148)

Spinach and Mushroom Pizza Pie (page 153)

Iron

An adequate intake of iron keeps you feeling energetic and healthy. Not having enough can lead to iron deficiency anemia, which can cause you to look pale and feel tired or run down. Getting enough iron is a particular concern for children, women, pregnant women, vegetarians and female athletes.

Iron comes in two forms, *heme* iron and *non-heme* iron. Heme iron, found in animal-based foods, is generally more easily absorbed than non-heme iron, which is found in plant-based foods.

Heme iron is found in beef, pork, poultry, lamb, fish (halibut, haddock, perch, salmon, shrimp, canned sardines, tuna) and eggs. Non-heme iron is found in cooked clams, oysters, beans, peas and lentils, pumpkin, sesame and squash seeds, iron-enriched breakfast cereals, tofu, enriched egg noodles and pasta, dried apricots, nuts, bread, oatmeal, wheat germ, canned beets, canned pumpkin, dried raisins, peaches, prunes and apricots.

To increase iron absorption:

❧ Eat heme-iron foods with plant-based (non-heme) foods. For example, add ground beef to chili, or chicken to pasta salad.

❧ Eat non-heme iron foods along with those rich in vitamin C. For example, eat bean salad with tomatoes, or breakfast cereal with strawberries or orange juice.

❧ Avoid coffee or tea between meals, since these beverages can interfere with iron absorption.

Iron-clad meals

Here's a list of recipes in this book rated "very high in" or "excellent source of" iron.

Big-Batch Bran Muffins (page 33)

Swiss Chard Frittata in a Pita (page 62)

Seafood Chowder (page 74)

Crockpot Beef Stew (page 105)

Meatloaf "Muffins" with Barbecue Sauce (page 109)

Veggie, Beef and Pasta Bake (page 114)

Creamy Bow-Tie Pasta with Chicken, Spinach and Peppers (page 126)

Hot 'n' Spicy Turkey Burgers (page 131)

Turkey Pot Pie with Biscuit Topping (page 134)

Crunchy Fish Burgers (page 137)

Pasta with White Clam Sauce (page 139)

Shrimp and Mussels with Couscous (page 142)

Spaghettini with Tuna, Olives and Capers (page 143)

Crowd-Pleasing Vegetarian Chili (page 147)

Fettuccine Carbonara (page 148)

Pasta with Roasted Vegetables and Goat Cheese (page 149)

Penne with Mushrooms and Spicy Tomato Sauce (page 151)

Rotini with Vegetable Tomato Sauce (page 152)

Spinach and Mushroom Pizza Pie (page 153)

Sodium

For some people, excessive sodium intake (from eating too much salt) can contribute to high blood pressure, a risk factor for heart disease and stroke.

Most of the sodium in our diet comes from processed foods such as pickled foods, cured or smoked meats, cold cuts, crackers, snack foods like chips and pretzels, salted nuts, powdered soup and sauce mixes, canned soup and broth, canned foods and fast foods such as pizza or fries.

To reduce your salt intake, watch out for processed foods and cut down on the salt you use in cooking and at the table. Instead of salt, try different flavorings such as herbs, spices, garlic, onions, lemon juice and vinegar. The simplest method may be just to taste your food before adding salt – chances are you'll find the food really doesn't need it!

Do you need vitamin pills?

If you eat a variety of foods based on *Canada's Food Guide to Healthy Eating* you probably don't require vitamin or mineral supplements. There are some cases, however, when they are helpful.

🎐 Infants who are exclusively breast-fed require a vitamin D supplement.

🎐 Individuals who have a limited exposure to sunlight, such as the elderly, may benefit from a vitamin D supplement.

🎐 Children or adults who don't eat milk products may need a calcium supplement.

🎐 Pregnant women and women of childbearing years can benefit from a multivitamin supplement that supplies folic acid, iron and calcium.

🎐 Elderly people who eat poorly can benefit from a multivitamin to reduce their risk of nutrient deficiencies and infections.

The important thing to remember is that supplements are not a substitute for healthy eating. They don't provide energy (calories), trace vitamins, fiber and other non-nutritive substances that we get from food. And a supplement does not provide the taste and enjoyment you get from food. Still, if you think you need a supplement, consult your dietitian or doctor.

Health note: Some supplements, particularly vitamins A or D, can build up to toxic levels if taken in excess. It is safer to take a multi-vitamin rather than single-nutrient supplements; be sure to follow the dose specified on the package.

Drinking and Dining

Water. Drinking about 8 cups (2 L) of water or non-alcoholic liquid – such as juice, lemonade, milk, soups and herbal teas – each day helps to satisfy your body's need for fluids. Watch out for beverages that are high in caffeine, however, since they cause your body to lose water. You can compensate by drinking more water or you can just choose decaffeinated beverages instead.

Alcohol. In moderation, alcohol can be part of a healthy diet. For most adults, that means having no more than one drink per day and no more than 7 drinks a week. Here, one drink is defined as 5 oz (148 mL) wine, one 12-oz (355 mL) bottle of beer or 1 1/2 oz (44 mL) liquor. Women who are pregnant (or trying to become pregnant) should avoid alcohol.

HEALTHY WEIGH OF LIFE

Having a healthy body weight is important to help you feel good and to protect your health. However, it's important to determine if you are at risk for any weight-related health problems before considering weight-loss efforts. Your weight may already be within a healthy range. Check your Body Mass Index (BMI) using the chart on page 175. You'll find that there's a whole range of weights for healthy bodies of any given height.

It's important to have realistic expectations about your size and shape and to take a healthy-eating, active-living and feeling-good-about-yourself approach to achieving a healthy weight.

MAKE THE MOVE TO
better HEALTH

If each day you are active for at least 30 minutes – either in one continuous workout or at intervals throughout the day – that should be enough to produce heart-healthy results and maintain a healthy weight. Being physically active will also help you feel more energetic, increase your bone mass and muscle strength, improve your self-esteem, help you cope better with stress and feel more relaxed.

Exercising needn't be a chore. Build enjoyable activities into your daily routine to keep you strong, fit and flexible. *Canada's Physical Activity Guide to Healthy Active Living* outlines ways you can get active your way, every day – for life! You can get a copy of this guide at your local health department or fitness center or on the Internet at *www.paguide.com.*

Find out more about healthy eating

You can find information about nutrition and healthy eating almost anywhere these days. Unfortunately, there is a lot of misinformation to sort through, so it's wise to find reliable sources of information.

You can begin your search with the Dietitians of Canada website *www.dietitians.ca* or the Canadian Health Network website *www.canadian-health-network.ca.*

If you need healthy eating information or personal advice about your diet, contact a Registered Dietitian.

To find a Registered Dietitian in your community, contact your local department of public health, community health center or hospital. You can also get a list of Registered Dietitians who work in private practice on the Dietitians of Canada website (see address above) or by calling the Consulting Dietitians Network at 1-888-901-7776.

Sensible steps to a healthy weight

* Remember that great bodies come in all shapes and sizes.

* Keep your body moving. Regular physical activity can help you attain and maintain a healthy weight and keeps you looking and feeling your best.

* Eat breakfast every day. People who eat breakfast regularly have healthier weights than those who do not.

* Listen to your body: eat when you are hungry and quit when you are full.

* Eat balanced meals and snacks that include plenty of fiber and not too much fat.

* If you need to lose weight, it should come off the way it went on – slowly! A healthy rate of weight loss is 1 to 2 lbs (500 g to 1 kg) per week.

* Avoid quick weight loss programs or supplements. Instead, focus on exercising more and improving overall food choices.

About the Nutrient Values in this book

Computer-assisted nutrient analysis of the recipes was performed by Info Access (1988) Inc., Don Mills, Ontario, using the Nutritional Accounting component of the CBORD Menu Management System. The nutrient database was the 1997 Canadian Nutrient File supplemented when necessary with documented data from reliable sources.

The analysis was based on:

• imperial measures and weights (except for foods typically packaged and used in metric quantity)

• the smaller number of servings when there was a range

• the smaller ingredient quantity when there was a range

• the first ingredient listed when there was a choice.

Unless otherwise stated, recipes were analyzed using canola vegetable oil, soft-tub margarine, 1% flavored yogurt, and 2% milk, buttermilk, plain yogurt and cottage cheese, and unenriched pasta. Calculations of meat and poultry recipes assumed that only the lean portion without skin was eaten. Salt was included only when a specific amount was given, and was not used when cooking pasta. Optional ingredients and garnishes in unspecified amounts were not included in the analysis.

Nutrient values were rounded to the nearest whole number for calories and sodium and to one decimal place for protein, fat, carbohydrate and fiber. Excellent and good sources of selected vitamins and minerals were also identified. According to the criteria for food labeling (Guide to Food Labeling and Advertising, Canadian Food Inspection Agency, Agriculture and Agri-Food Canada, March 1996) a serving supplying 15% of the Recommended Daily Intake (RDI) of a vitamin or mineral (30% for vitamin C) is described as a good source. One supplying 25% of the RDI (50% for vitamin C) is described as an excellent source. A serving containing at least 2 grams of dietary fiber is described as a moderate source, a serving containing at least 4 grams of dietary fiber is described as a high source, and a serving containing at least 6 grams of dietary fiber as a very high source.

Food Guide servings

Canada's Food Guide to Healthy Eating contains daily serving recommendations for foods from four groups (Grain Products, Vegetables & Fruit, Milk Products, and Meat & Alternatives) and displays serving sizes for selected items. The number of *Food Guide* servings contributed by each recipe portion was calculated using customized software developed by Info Access. Serving sizes for ingredients not specifically mentioned in the *Food Guide* were approximated with reference to the serving size and nutrient contribution of other foods in the same food group. Ranges are provided in the *Food Guide* for Meats & Alternatives. In assigning the number of servings provided by a recipe, 2 to 4 oz (50 to 100 g) meat, 1 egg or 1/2 cup (125 mL) beans and lentils were each counted as one Meat & Alternatives serving.

The number of servings for Milk Products and Meat & Alternatives were rounded to quarter servings, while those for Grain Products and Vegetables & Fruit were rounded to half servings. The nutrient contribution of the specific foods in the recipe was considered when rounding these assignments.

GETTING OFF TO A GREAT START

Start your day th

Break your fast with a nutrient-packed meal that provides about 25% of your daily energy and nutritional needs.

Try to include foods from at least three of the four food groups in *Canada's Food Guide to Healthy Eating* (see page 176).

A balanced breakfast ca be as fast and easy as a bowl of cereal with milk and a glass of juice, or

BREAKFAST *Breaking the fast*

The recipes in this section are perfect for people who don't have much time for breakfast. Many of these recipes can be made ahead of time (muffins, for example), while others (such as breakfast shakes) can be made quickly and taken with you as you dash out the door. Some recipes are there purely for your enjoyment – on those all-too-rare occasions when you have some time to linger over breakfast.

Having something to eat soon after you wake provides the energy and nutrients you need to take on the physical and mental challenges of the day ahead.

After eight or more hours without eating, your blood-sugar level is low. Eating soon after waking satisfies hunger but also helps improve concentration and mental alertness.

Eating breakfast has been shown to help improve learning and school performance in children.

Breakfast is the meal that's most often missed.

People who skip breakfast rarely make up for the nutrients they missed at breakfast later in the day.

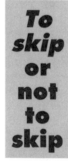

To skip or not to skip

Children and adults who eat breakfast on a regular basis have been found to have healthier weights – and a healthier lifestyle than those who skip breakfast.

What if you don't feel like eating when you first wake up?

If you don't feel hungry when you wake up, it may be that you ate too much before going to sleep. In this case, you may want to try eating more food earlier in the day, when your body is more active.

But if you simply can't face food first thing in the morning, try easing into it. A small nutritious snack mid-morning is better than having nothing at all.

balanced way

a slice of pizza with a glass of milk and a piece of fruit, or a microwave-cooked egg with toast and a glass of juice.

Getting children to eat breakfast regularly sets the stage for a lifetime of healthy eating habits.

Parents can set a good example by eating a balanced breakfast with their children whenever possible.

WHAT about caffeine?

Moderate consumption of caffeine has not been proven to cause health problems. According to Health Canada's nutrition recommendations, intakes of 400 to 450 mg of caffeine a day (3 to 4 cups of coffee or tea) are okay. Be sure that beverages containing caffeine don't displace more nutritious drinks such as milk, juice or water.

STIMULATING CONTENT

Caffeine contained in common beverages
(per 6 oz [175 mL])

	Caffeine
Coffee, automatic percolated	72 to 144 mg
Coffee, filter drip	108 to 180 mg
Coffee, instant, regular	60 to 90 mg
Coffee, instant, decaffeinated	less than 6 mg
Tea, weak	18 to 24 mg
Tea, strong	78 to 108 mg
Hot cocoa	6 to 30 mg
Cola soft drink, half 12 oz (355 mL) can	14 to 32 mg

*Source: Caffeine Issue Paper. Health Protection Branch, Health and Welfare Canada, 1992

Fast-and-easy energizers to eat at home or on the go

- *fruity yogurt shake with a bran, oatmeal or other whole grain muffin*
- *peanut butter and banana sandwich and a glass of milk*
- *toasted whole grain English muffin with a slice of cheese and a piece of fruit*
- *bran cereal with milk and berries*
- *cereal bar, yogurt and a container of juice*
- *bag of mixed dry cereals, nuts and dried fruit and a container of milk*
- *bagel with Cheddar cheese and vegetable juice cocktail*
- *poached egg on a bun with a glass of juice*

Better breakfast

Breakfast helps increase overall nutrient intake – especially when the meal includes nutrient-rich choices.

Eating a breakfast that's low in fat and high in fiber is a great way to start your day.

Good breakfast choices include: whole wheat, bran and oat cereals; whole grain bread or bagels; fresh, canned or dried fruit; milk products; and eggs.

Eating on the run

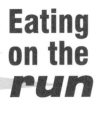

When you have things to do and places to go, it's often difficult to have a complete breakfast in one sitting. That's okay – as long as you eat a variety of healthy foods throughout the morning.

If schedules are too hectic for a sit-down meal it's a good idea to pack a breakfast that can be eaten on the run.

SERVES 1

Dairy Farmers of Canada [P]

Sunny Orange Shake

MAKES 1 1/4 CUPS (300 mL)

Quick Shake

Once a week, 12-year-old Amelia Roblin gets up early to treat her dad to this quick and delicious smoothie. She uses 1/2 cup (125 mL) milk, one 6-oz (175 g) container flavored yogurt and 1/2 cup (125 mL) fruit, and mixes everything up in a blender. The flavor combinations are endless: banana yogurt and canned mandarin oranges; peach yogurt and strawberries; lemon yogurt and frozen blueberries; strawberry yogurt and banana; and vanilla yogurt and canned peaches.

3/4 cup	vanilla-flavored lower-fat yogurt	175 mL
2 tbsp	skim milk powder	25 mL
1/2 cup	orange juice	125 mL

1. In a blender combine yogurt, skim milk powder and orange juice; blend until smooth.

Complete the meal
Pour this shake into a travel mug and enjoy it in transit, accompanied by a whole-grain bagel, muffin or a cereal bar.

TIP

Shakes are a fast and easy way to increase your intake of milk and fruit. This shake is especially suited to people who like their shakes smooth – without any "bits" in it.

Nutrition Facts

Skim milk powder adds extra thickness and boosts the calcium content of this shake to 353 mg per serving. It is also low in fat.

food guide servings

GRAIN PRODUCTS	VEGETABLES & FRUIT
	1
1 1/2	
MILK PRODUCTS	MEAT & ALTERNATIVES

nutrient analysis

PER SERVING			
Calories	262	Carbohydrate	50.8 g
Protein	10.8 g	Dietary Fiber	0.4 g
Fat	1.9 g	Sodium	147 mg

Excellent source of calcium, vitamin C, riboflavin, folacin and vitamin B_{12}. **Good** source of zinc and thiamin.

Ann Merritt
TORONTO, ON

P

SERVES 2

Banana-Berry Wake-Up Shake

MAKES ABOUT 3 1/4 CUPS (800 mL)

Frozen sliced bananas work well in these shakes and help make them creamy. When bananas start to get brown, pop them in the freezer and take out as needed.

1	banana	1
1 cup	fresh or frozen berries (any combination)	250 mL
1 cup	milk *or* vanilla-flavored soy beverage	250 mL
3/4 cup	lower-fat yogurt (vanilla or other flavor that complements berries)	175 mL

TIP

The vanilla yogurt used in these shake recipes (and in SUNNY ORANGE SHAKE, see page 32) is higher in carbohydrate than most other yogurts. People with diabetes may want to choose a lower-carbohydrate brand.

1. In a blender liquefy fruit with a small amount of the milk. Add remaining milk and yogurt; blend until smooth. If shake is too thick, add extra milk or soy beverage to achieve desired consistency.

Complete the meal

Enjoy this shake with PUMPKIN RAISIN MUFFINS (see recipe, page 35) or ORANGE-APRICOT OATMEAL SCONES (see recipe, page 36).

Nutrition Facts

These shakes are packed with bone-building calcium. People who are allergic to milk or who are lactose intolerant can substitute a calcium-fortified soy beverage and soy yogurt.

Make Ahead

Make these shakes the night before and you'll be ready for a quick morning meal to go.

food guide servings

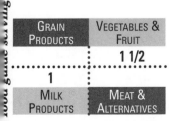

GRAIN PRODUCTS	VEGETABLES & FRUIT
	1 1/2
1	
MILK PRODUCTS	MEAT & ALTERNATIVES

nutrient analysis

PER SERVING			
Calories	234	Carbohydrate	43.8 g
Protein	8.7 g	Dietary Fiber	3.2 g
Fat	3.8 g	Sodium	114 mg

Excellent source of calcium, riboflavin, vitamin B$_6$ and B$_{12}$. **Good** source of vitamin C and folacin. **Moderate** source of dietary fiber.

MAKES 1

Shauna Ratner, RDN
VANCOUVER, BC [P]

Banana Bread

PREHEAT OVEN TO 350° F (180° C)
9- BY 5-INCH (2 L) BAKING PAN, GREASED

"We make this banana bread all the time at home," Shauna says. *It is delicious with a handful of fresh blueberries, frozen cranberries or chocolate chips added to the recipe.*

1 1/4 cups	all-purpose flour	300 mL
1 tsp	baking soda	5 mL
1/2 tsp	baking powder	2 mL
3/4 cup	granulated sugar	175 mL
1	egg	1
1	egg white	1
1/4 cup	lower-fat plain yogurt	50 mL
1/4 cup	vegetable oil	50 mL
1 tsp	vanilla	5 mL
1 cup	mashed ripe bananas (about 2 to 3 medium)	250 mL

Nutrition Facts

Substitute up to 1/2 cup (125 mL) whole wheat flour for all-purpose flour if you have it. If the bananas are super-ripe you can decrease sugar to 1/2 cup (125 mL).

Make Ahead

Make an extra loaf and freeze for another day or freeze well-wrapped individual slices of banana bread and pull them out as needed to add to lunch bags.

1. In a bowl sift together flour, baking soda and baking powder. Set aside.

2. In a large mixing bowl, blend sugar, egg, egg white, yogurt, oil and vanilla. Blend in bananas. Add dry ingredients; mix until just combined. Pour batter into prepared pan. Bake in preheated oven for 1 hour or until a tester inserted in center of loaf comes out clean.

complete the meal

Serve with orange or grapefruit juice and a quick scrambled egg (see recipe, page 40).

Variation

To make a muffin version of this recipe, spoon batter into 12 greased muffin cups. Bake at 350° F (180° C) for 18 to 22 minutes or until firm to the touch.

food guide servings

GRAIN PRODUCTS	VEGETABLES & FRUIT
1/2	
MILK PRODUCTS	MEAT & ALTERNATIVES

nutrient analysis

PER SLICE (12 SLICES PER LOAF)			
Calories	165	Carbohydrate	27.4 g
Protein	2.6 g	Dietary Fiber	0.7 g
Fat	5.3 g	Sodium	122 mg

PUMPKIN RAISIN MUFFINS (PAGE 35) • BANANA-BERRY WAKE-UP SHAKE (PAGE 31) ➤

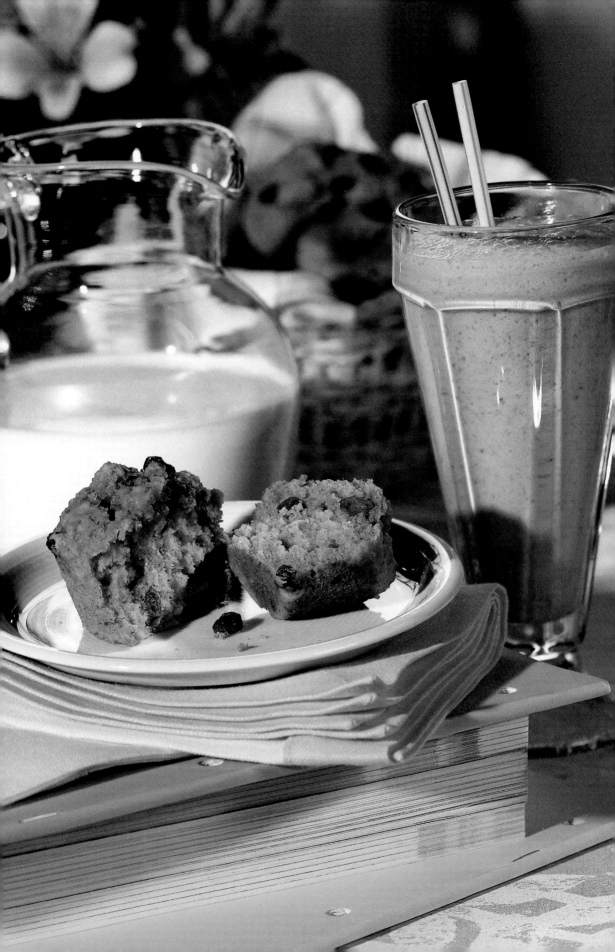

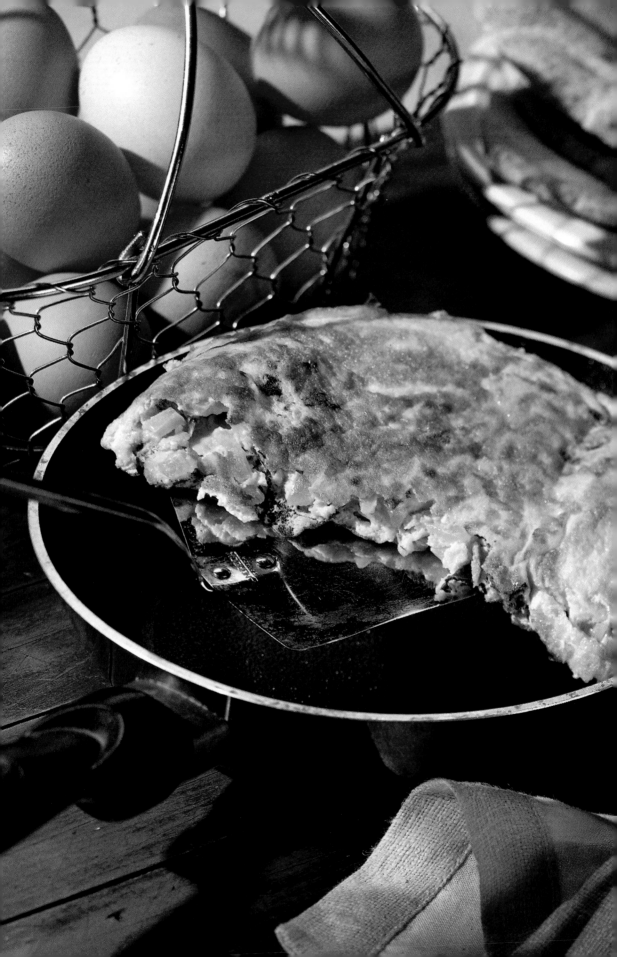

MAKES 24   Big-Batch Bran Muffins

Susanne Stark
Post Cereals
TORONTO, ON

P

PREHEAT OVEN TO 375° F (190° C)
TWO 12-CUP MUFFIN TINS, GREASED OR PAPER-LINED

TIP

This batter can be prepared and stored for up to 2 weeks in the refrigerator. Pour batter into prepared muffin tins and bake as needed. Or you can bake the whole batch and keep extras in the freezer.

Sour milk can be used instead of buttermilk. To prepare, combine 3 tbsp (45 mL) lemon juice or white vinegar with 4 cups (1 L) milk and let stand for 5 minutes.

Nutrition Facts

Eating bran muffins for breakfast is a great way to get more fiber into your day. Wheat bran promotes regularity and a healthy digestive system.

5 cups	all-purpose flour	1.25 L
5 1/2 cups	100% bran cereal	1.375 L
2 cups	packed brown sugar	500 mL
1 cup	chopped dates or raisins	250 mL
1 tbsp	baking soda	15 mL
1 tbsp	cinnamon	15 mL
4 cups	buttermilk *or* sour milk (see Tip, at left)	1 L
1 cup	vegetable oil	250 mL
4	eggs	4

1. In a large bowl, combine flour, cereal, brown sugar, dates, baking soda and cinnamon.

2. In another large bowl, mix together buttermilk, oil and eggs. Stir into dry ingredients and mix until moistened.

3. Spoon batter into muffin cups, generously filling to the top. Bake in preheated oven for 25 to 30 minutes or until golden brown. Cool in pans for 5 minutes; remove muffins. Cool on a wire rack. Store in airtight containers; freeze, if desired.

Complete the meal
Pack these muffins along with a BANANA-BERRY WAKE-UP SHAKE (see recipe, page 31) for a quick meal to go.

food guide servings

GRAIN PRODUCTS	VEGETABLES & FRUIT
2	
MILK PRODUCTS	MEAT & ALTERNATIVES

nutrient analysis

PER MUFFIN			
Calories	331	Carbohydrate	57.2 g
Protein	7.0 g	Dietary Fiber	6.8 g
Fat	10.8 g	Sodium	334 mg

Excellent source of thiamin and iron. **Good** source of riboflavin, niacin, vitamin B6, folacin and zinc. **Very high** in dietary fiber.

◄ SWISS CHARD FRITTATA (PAGE 62)

MAKES 24

Cornmeal Muffins

Bev Callaghan, RD

P

TIP

Keep a supply of these muffins frozen in airtight containers until needed for breakfast, lunch or snacks. Defrost in the microwave for breakfast or pop into a lunch bag directly from the freezer; they'll defrost by the time lunch rolls around.

Sour milk can be used instead of buttermilk. To prepare, combine 3 tbsp (45 mL) lemon juice or white vinegar with 4 cups (1 L) milk and let stand for 5 minutes.

Nutrition Facts
Fruit punch and flavored drinks don't deliver the same nutrients as fresh fruit juice or juice from concentrate.

4 cups	all-purpose flour	1 L
2 cups	cornmeal	500 mL
3/4 cup	granulated sugar	175 mL
2 tbsp	baking powder	25 mL
2 tsp	baking soda	10 mL
1/2 tsp	salt	2 mL
4 cups	buttermilk *or* sour milk (see Tip, at left)	1 L
1/2 cup	vegetable oil	125 mL
3	eggs	3

1. In a bowl combine flour, cornmeal, all but 2 tsp (10 mL) of the sugar, baking powder, baking soda and salt.

2. In a separate bowl, whisk together buttermilk, oil and eggs. Add to dry ingredients; stir just until combined.

3. Spoon into muffin cups. Sprinkle with remaining sugar. Bake in preheated oven for 18 to 22 minutes or until firm to the touch.

Complete the meal
Have with a SUNNY ORANGE SHAKE (see recipe, page 30) for breakfast or pack in a lunch bag with a thermos of FAST CHILI (see recipe, page 106) and a container of milk or yogurt.

food guide servings

GRAIN PRODUCTS	VEGETABLES & FRUIT
1 1/2	

MILK PRODUCTS	MEAT & ALTERNATIVES

nutrient analysis

PER MUFFIN			
Calories	209	Carbohydrate	33.4 g
Protein	5.2 g	Dietary Fiber	1.2 g
Fat	5.9 g	Sodium	261 mg

MAKES 24 Pumpkin Raisin Muffins

Tracy Nash, RD
PRINCE ALBERT, AB

P

PREHEAT OVEN TO 375° F (190° C)
TWO 12-CUP MUFFIN TINS, GREASED OR PAPER-LINED

Nutrition Facts

Eating dark-colored vegetables and fruit – such as pumpkins, cantaloupe, carrots or red bell peppers – is a great way to boost your intake of vitamin A and beta carotene.

Sour milk can be used instead of buttermilk. To prepare, combine 4 tsp (20 mL) lemon juice or white vinegar with 2 cups (500 mL) milk and let stand for 5 minutes.

Make Ahead

These muffins freeze well, so make up an extra batch and store in the freezer in an airtight container or freezer bag until needed.

mplete the meal

Serve with juice or fruit, a glass of milk, and a quick-cooked egg (see page 41).

2 cups	whole wheat flour	500 mL
1 1/2 cups	all-purpose flour	375 mL
1 cup	granulated sugar	250 mL
4 tsp	baking powder	20 mL
1 tsp	baking soda	5 mL
1 tbsp	cinnamon	15 mL
1 tsp	ground nutmeg	5 mL
1 tsp	ground ginger	5 mL
1/4 tsp	salt	1 mL
1 1/2 cups	raisins	375 mL
1	can (14 oz [398 mL]) pumpkin purée (not pie filling)	1
1/2 cup	vegetable oil	125 mL
2 cups	buttermilk *or* sour milk (see Tip, at left)	500 mL
3	eggs	3

1. In a large bowl, combine whole wheat flour, all-purpose flour, sugar, baking powder, baking soda, cinnamon, nutmeg, ginger, salt and raisins.

2. In a separate bowl, blend together pumpkin, oil, buttermilk and eggs.

3. Make a large well in center of dry ingredients; pour in wet ingredients all at once. Gently fold together until just combined.

4. Spoon batter into muffin tins. Bake in preheated oven for 18 to 22 minutes or until firm to the touch.

food guide servings

GRAIN PRODUCTS	VEGETABLES & FRUIT
1	1/2

MILK PRODUCTS	MEAT & ALTERNATIVES

nutrient analysis

PER MUFFIN			
Calories	191	Carbohydrate	32.6 g
Protein	4.2 g	Dietary Fiber	2.3 g
Fat	5.7 g	Sodium	148 mg

Excellent source of vitamin A.
Moderate source of dietary fiber.

MAKES 12

Bev Callaghan, RD   P

Orange-Apricot Oatmeal Scones

PREHEAT OVEN TO 375° F (190° C) • BAKING SHEET, GREASED

2 cups	all-purpose flour	500 mL
1 1/2 cups	quick rolled oats	375 mL
1/4 cup	granulated sugar	50 mL
1 tbsp	baking powder	15 mL
2 tsp	grated orange zest	10 mL
1/2 tsp	baking soda	2 mL
1/4 tsp	salt	1 mL
6 tbsp	butter	90 mL
1/2 cup	chopped apricots	125 mL
1 cup	buttermilk *or* sour milk (see Tip, at left)	250 mL
	Milk	

Make Ahead

These freeze well, so make up an extra batch and store them in an airtight container or freezer bags and freeze. Take out as needed for breakfast, lunch or snacks.

1. In a bowl combine flour, oats, all but 1 tsp (5 mL) of the sugar, baking powder, orange zest, baking soda and salt. Using a fork or pastry blender, cut in butter until mixture resembles coarse crumbs. Stir in apricots. Add buttermilk; stir until mixture is just combined.

2. On a lightly floured surface, knead dough gently about 4 or 5 times. Divide dough into 3 pieces. Shape each piece into a round about 1 inch (2.5 cm) thick. Transfer to baking sheet.

3. Cut each round into four quarters. Brush tops with milk; sprinkle with reserved sugar. Bake in preheated oven for 20 to 25 minutes or until lightly browned.

Variation

For a change, substitute 1/2 cup (125 mL) dried cranberries, dates, raisins or currants for the apricots.

Sour milk can be used instead of buttermilk. To prepare, combine 2 tsp (10 mL) lemon juice or white vinegar with 1 cup (250 mL) milk and let stand for 5 minutes.

complete the meal
Try these scones with a glass of milk and a piece of fruit. They also taste great with a SUNNY ORANGE SHAKE (see recipe, page 30).

food guide servings

GRAIN PRODUCTS	VEGETABLES & FRUIT
1 1/2	
MILK PRODUCTS	MEAT & ALTERNATIVES

nutrient analysis

PER SCONE			
Calories	205	Carbohydrate	31.8 g
Protein	4.7 g	Dietary Fiber	2.4 g
Fat	6.8 g	Sodium	242 mg

Moderate source of dietary fiber.

Bev Callaghan, RD

SERVES 1

P

Creamy Microwave Oatmeal

1/2 cup	water	125 mL
1/2 cup	milk *or* soy beverage	125 mL
1/8 tsp	salt	0.5 mL
2 tbsp	raisins	25 mL
1 tsp	wheat bran	5 mL
1/2 cup	quick rolled oats	125 mL
1/4 tsp	cinnamon	1 mL
	Brown sugar *or* maple syrup	
	Milk	

1. In a 4-cup (1 L) microwave-safe bowl, combine water, milk, salt, raisins and bran. Microwave on High for 2 minutes. Stir in oats and cinnamon; microwave on High for 3 to 4 minutes, stirring at 1-minute intervals until oatmeal has thickened. Cover and let stand for 1 minute. Serve with brown sugar or maple syrup, and milk.

Complete the meal

To add some vitamin C to your meal, serve this oatmeal with half a grapefruit or a glass of orange juice.

TIP

This is the oatmeal Bev enjoys most weekday mornings (although she's also partial to BREAKFAST MUESLI TO GO [see recipe, page 39]). She credits her father for introducing her to the merits of having hot cereal for breakfast.

This recipe is easily multiplied to serve 2, 3 or 4 people. To make in a saucepan, combine water, milk, salt, raisins and bran. Bring to a boil over medium heat. While stirring constantly, add oats and cinnamon; reduce heat to low and simmer, covered, for 3 to 4 minutes.

Nutrition Facts

Here's an easy way to boost your calcium intake: When preparing any hot cereal, substitute milk for half of the water that is called for in the package directions.
This breakfast provides both soluble fiber from oatmeal and insoluble fiber from wheat bran. Including both types of fiber in your daily meals is beneficial to your long-term good health.

food guide servings

GRAIN PRODUCTS	VEGETABLES & FRUIT
1 1/2	
1/2	
MILK PRODUCTS	MEAT & ALTERNATIVES

nutrient analysis

PER SERVING			
Calories	282	Carbohydrate	50.7 g
Protein	11.4 g	Dietary Fiber	6.0 g
Fat	5.1 g	Sodium	355 mg

Good source of calcium, iron, zinc, thiamin and riboflavin. **Very high** in dietary fiber.

SERVES 14

Muesli Mix

Stefa Katamay, RD
DEEP RIVER, ON

TIP

This is Stefa's favorite break-fast food – her kids and husband Bruce love it too! She varies it to taste with different types of fruit and berries, depending on the season.

Food Fast

Take a small container of this muesli to work or school and combine with yogurt for a quick snack. It's also great for camping, backpacking, and canoe trips.

Nutrition Facts

This high-fiber cereal can help keep you regular. To add even more fiber and additional nutrients, try it with peaches or blueberries.

4 cups	quick rolled oats	1 L
1/2 cup	flax seeds	125 mL
1/2 cup	wheat germ	125 mL
1/2 cup	oat bran	125 mL
1/2 cup	wheat bran	125 mL
1 cup	dried cranberries	250 mL

1. Mix all ingredients together and pour into an air-tight container. Store in a cool, dry place.

Complete the meal

For a balanced break-fast, mix this cereal in a bowl with 3/4 cup (175 mL) plain yogurt and 1/2 cup (125 mL) fresh or canned fruit. Add honey or maple syrup to taste.

food guide servings

GRAIN PRODUCTS	VEGETABLES & FRUIT
1	
MILK PRODUCTS	MEAT & ALTERNATIVES

nutrient analysis

PER 1/2 CUP (125 ML) SERVING			
Calories	169	Carbohydrate	29.5 g
Protein	6.7 g	Dietary Fiber	5.6 g
Fat	4.2 g	Sodium	6 mg

Good source of iron, zinc, thiamin and folacin.
High in dietary fiber.

SERVES 2 — Breakfast Muesli to Go

Renée Crompton, RD
OTTAWA, ON   P

This is a complete breakfast for people who have to rush in the morning. Renée says, "it has the best consistency and taste if made the night before." She divides it into two sealable containers and leaves room to add some banana.

1 cup	large-flake or 3-minute oats (not instant)	250 mL
1 cup	lower-fat plain yogurt	250 mL
1/2 cup	milk	125 mL
2 tbsp	liquid honey *or* maple syrup	25 mL
1 cup	assorted berries (fresh or frozen)	250 mL
1	large banana, sliced	1

1. In a plastic container, combine oats, yogurt, milk and honey; gently fold in berries. Add banana before serving or add to sealable container before taking muesli on the go.

Complete the meal

This is a filling breakfast. A glass of juice goes down nicely.

TIP

For variety, try different types of yogurt and fresh fruits in season. If using vanilla or fruit-flavored yogurt, omit the honey.

Nutrition Facts

A single serving of this muesli is very high in fiber and provides about half your recommended daily intake for vitamin C and calcium.

food guide servings

GRAIN PRODUCTS	VEGETABLES & FRUIT
1 1/2	1 1/2
1	
MILK PRODUCTS	MEAT & ALTERNATIVES

nutrient analysis

PER SERVING			
Calories	423	Carbohydrate	79.2 g
Protein	16.0 g	Dietary Fiber	7.9 g
Fat	6.8 g	Sodium	117 mg

Excellent source of calcium, zinc, vitamin C, thiamin, riboflavin, vitamin B_6 and B_{12}. **Good** source of iron, niacin and folacin. **Very high** in dietary fiber.

SERVES 2

Finnish Apple Pancake

Kimberly Green, RD
THUNDER BAY, ON

PREHEAT OVEN TO 425° F (220° C)
8-INCH (2 L) SQUARE BAKING PAN, GREASED

According to Kimberly, "this is an easy recipe for a special breakfast and it reflects the Finnish heritage around the Thunder Bay area."

2 cups	thinly sliced apples, peeled and cored	500 mL
1 tbsp	butter, melted	15 mL
3	eggs	3
1/2 cup	milk	125 mL
1/3 cup	all-purpose flour	75 mL
1/4 tsp	baking powder	1 mL
1/8 tsp	salt	0.5 mL

Topping

1/2 tsp	cinnamon	2 mL
1 tbsp	granulated sugar	15 mL

1. Place apples and butter in pan; toss to coat. Bake in preheated oven for 5 minutes.

2. Meanwhile, in a small bowl, whisk together eggs, milk, flour, baking powder and salt until smooth. Set aside.

3. Topping: In another small bowl, combine cinnamon and sugar. Set aside.

4. Pour egg mixture over cooked apples; sprinkle evenly with topping. Bake for 15 to 20 minutes or until pancake is puffed and golden brown. Serve immediately with maple syrup or your favorite fruit preserves.

Quick Scrambled Eggs For One

Using a microwave is a great way to teach children how to prepare their own meals.

In a microwave-safe bowl, whisk 2 eggs with 2 tbsp (25 mL) milk and salt and pepper to taste. Cover with plastic wrap, leaving a small steam vent. Microwave on Medium-High for 1 minute 30 seconds to 1 minute 45 seconds, stirring several times during cooking. Cover and let stand for 30 seconds to 1 minute before serving. Eggs will look slightly moist at first but will finish cooking while covered.

complete the meal
This is a complete breakfast but having it with a glass of milk will increase your calcium intake. A serving of fruit or juice adds vitamin C.

food guide servings

GRAIN PRODUCTS	VEGETABLES & FRUIT
1	1
1/4	1
MILK PRODUCTS	MEAT & ALTERNATIVES

nutrient analysis

PER SERVING			
Calories	357	Carbohydrate	42.7 g
Protein	13.8 g	Dietary Fiber	3.3 g
Fat	14.9 g	Sodium	359 mg

Excellent source of riboflavin and vitamin B₁₂. **Good** source of iron, vitamin A, niacin and folacin. **Moderate** source of dietary fiber.

MAKES 8 | Fiber-Full Bran Pancakes

Louise J. Vautour
POINTE DU CHENE, NB

These flavorful pancakes can help boost your fiber intake. They taste wonderful with maple syrup or fruit preserves.

Nutrition Facts
Wheat germ is a source of vitamin E. It's easy to add it to muffins and pancakes.

3/4 cup	whole wheat flour	175 mL
1/2 cup	bran flakes cereal, crushed	125 mL
1/4 cup	wheat germ	50 mL
1 1/2 tsp	baking powder	7 mL
1/8 tsp	salt	0.5 mL
1 cup	milk	250 mL
1	egg	1
1	egg white	1
1 tbsp	vegetable oil	15 mL

1. In a medium bowl, combine flour, bran flakes, wheat germ, baking powder and salt. Set aside.

2. In a small bowl, blend together milk, egg, egg white and oil; stir into bran mixture until combined. For each pancake, pour about 1/4 cup (50 mL) batter onto nonstick griddle or frying pan. Cook, turning once, for about 1 to 2 minutes per side or until golden.

Quick-Cooked Egg
Break an egg into a small microwave-safe bowl or ramekin; pierce yolk with a fork. Cover with plastic wrap, leaving part open for venting. Microwave at Medium-High for 45 seconds to 1 minute or until desired consistency is reached. Let stand 1 to 2 minutes without removing the plastic wrap.

Complete the meal
These pancakes are delicious with a glass of juice or 1/2 cup of fresh or canned fruit.

food guide servings

GRAIN PRODUCTS	VEGETABLES & FRUIT
1 1/2	
1/4	1/2
MILK PRODUCTS	MEAT & ALTERNATIVES

nutrient analysis

PER 2 PANCAKES			
Calories	208	Carbohydrate	28.8 g
Protein	9.8 g	Dietary Fiber	4.8 g
Fat	7.0 g	Sodium	285 mg

Excellent source of thiamin. **Good** source of iron, zinc, riboflavin, niacin and folacin. **High** in dietary fiber.

SERVES 2

Canadian Egg Marketing Agency

Individual Salsa Fresca Omelettes

Food Fast

With all the ingredients on hand, this recipe is quick to prepare and serve for breakfast, lunch or dinner. If you don't have time to make the salsa, use a commercially prepared salsa instead.

Make Ahead

Prepare the salsa the night before; put in an airtight container and store in the fridge.

Use about 1/2 cup (125 mL) salsa per omelette. The extra 1 cup (250 mL) salsa can be used in HURRY-UP FILL-ME-UP BURRITOS (see recipe, page 61) or as a dip for baked tortilla chips or Pita Crisps (see recipe, page 48).

Salsa Fresca

1 cup	diced seeded tomatoes	250 mL
1 cup	diced cucumber	250 mL
1/3 cup	chopped red onions	75 mL
1/4 cup	chopped fresh cilantro or parsley	50 mL
2 tbsp	lime juice	25 mL
	Salt and pepper to taste	

Omelettes

4	eggs	4
1 tbsp	water	15 mL
	Salt and pepper to taste	
1 tsp	butter *or* vegetable oil	5 mL

1. Salsa: In a bowl combine tomatoes, cucumber, red onions, cilantro, lime juice, salt and pepper. Let stand 10 minutes. Drain well.

2. Omelette: In a bowl, beat together eggs, water, salt and pepper. In a small 8-inch (20 cm) nonstick skillet over medium-high heat, melt 1/2 tsp (2 mL) butter. Making one omelette at a time, pour half of egg mixture into pan. As eggs begin to set at edges, use a spatula to gently push cooked portions to the center, tilting pan to allow uncooked egg to flow into empty spaces.

Complete the meal

Serve with whole grain toast, in a pita pocket or wrapped up in a whole wheat flour tortilla. Round out the meal with a glass of milk.

Variation

Dress up your omelette with chopped ham and green onions, shredded cheese or diced leftover cooked potatoes.

nutrient analysis

3. When egg is almost set on the surface but still looks moist, fill half the omelette with some of the Salsa Fresca. Slip spatula under unfilled side, fold over filling and slide omelette onto plate. Top with additional Salsa Fresca. Repeat with remaining egg mixture.

food guide servings

Grain Products	Vegetables & Fruit
	1
	1
Milk Products	Meat & Alternatives

PER OMELETTE WITH 1/2 CUP (125 mL) SALSA FRESCA			
Calories	185	Carbohydrate	5.9 g
Protein	13.2 g	Dietary Fiber	0.9 g
Fat	12.0 g	Sodium	150 mg

Excellent source of riboflavin and vitamin B_{12}. **Good** source of vitamin A and folacin.

SERVES 4

Canadian Egg
Marketing Agency [P]

Overnight Broccoli and Cheese Strata

9-INCH (2.5 L) CASSEROLE, GREASED

2 cups	chopped fresh broccoli or asparagus	500 mL
4 cups	whole-wheat bread (preferably stale), cubed	1 L
2 cups	shredded Swiss or Cheddar cheese	500 mL
4	eggs	4
2 cups	milk	500 mL
1/2 to 1 tsp	dry mustard	2 to 5 mL
	Cayenne pepper to taste (optional)	

1. In a pot of boiling water, cook broccoli just until tender-crisp; drain and pat dry. Set aside.

2. Place bread cubes in casserole dish. Add cheese and broccoli; gently toss together.

3. In a bowl, beat together eggs, milk, mustard and, if using, cayenne pepper; pour evenly over bread mixture. Cover and refrigerate for 2 hours or overnight.

4. Preheat oven to 350° F (180° C). Bake for 50 to 60 minutes or until golden brown and just set in center. Let stand for 3 to 4 minutes before serving.

TIP

This is a wonderful meal to make ahead for a special breakfast or brunch.

Frozen broccoli can easily be used in place of fresh broccoli. Place frozen broccoli in a microwave-safe bowl, cover and microwave on High for 2 minutes. Drain, pat dry and proceed with recipe.

Nutrition Facts

This meal provides an incredible 763 mg calcium per serving. It also provides fiber and many essential nutrients. Since it is relatively high in fat, balance the rest of your day with lower-fat foods.

Complete the meal

This is a fabulous four-food-group meal. Serve with a glass of fruit or vegetable juice, if desired.

food guide servings

GRAIN PRODUCTS	VEGETABLES & FRUIT
1	1
1 1/2	1
MILK PRODUCTS	MEAT & ALTERNATIVES

nutrient analysis

PER SERVING			
Calories	435	Carbohydrate	25.6 g
Protein	30.5 g	Dietary Fiber	3.9 g
Fat	23.9 g	Sodium	444 mg

Excellent source of calcium, zinc, vitamin C, A, riboflavin, niacin, folacin and vitamin B$_{12}$. **Good** source of iron. **Moderate** source of dietary fiber.

QUICK MEALS AND SNACKS

SNACKS *can be part of* *healthy eating*

The recipes in this section are great for those busy days when you get home and need a quick bite before dashing out again. Some recipes make enough appetizers to feed a crowd. Others are perfect for after school or work. Many recipes are suitable for packing into lunch bags and eating on the run.

Nutritious snacks help boost energy levels. Eating a number of small meals throughout the day helps to manage blood sugar levels and aid with weight control.

Skipping meals or going for long periods without food can lead to poor nutrition. Such habits may also encourage impulse eating or overeating later in the day, which can lead to weight gain.

Snack on foods from each of the four foods groups described in *Canada's Food Guide to Healthy Eating* for essential vitamins, minerals and fiber.

Not *all* snacks are created equal

Combine high-carbohydrate snacks (such as bagels, breads, cereal, fruit or vegetables) with protein-rich foods (such as milk, cheese, yogurt, meat, fish, poultry, eggs, peanut butter, nuts, seeds, beans or lentils) to keep you feeling satisfied longer.

Higher-fat snacks such as doughnuts, croissants, chips, chocolate bars, rich cookies, French fries or other deep-fried foods should be eaten in moderation.

Choose snacks that won't harm your teeth. Sticky sweets, dried fruits or other foods that are high in sugar or starch can cause cavities if eaten alone. Enjoy these foods with meals and, whenever possible, brush afterwards.

Keep *healthy snacks* close at hand

Nutritious snacking is easy if you keep healthy non-perishable snacks in your knapsack, briefcase, car or at work. Dry cereals, fig bars, whole grain crackers, cereal bars, dried fruit, nuts or seeds, individual containers of pudding or fruit, juice and water all keep well.

If you have access to a refrigerator at work, stock it with individual containers of yogurt, milk, cheese, and vegetable or fruit juices.

Good snack foods to keep around the house include fruit, vegetables, juice, pita bread, bagels, crackers, bread sticks, yogurt, milk, cheese, muffins, dry cereals, bean dips, hummus, peanut butter, nuts and seeds.

Make quick *meals-to-go*

Put together fast meals that can be heated up quickly in the microwave. Include last night's leftovers or a mixture of fresh foods. Try pasta dishes, canned beans, pizza, tortillas or burritos or the lunch-box meals found on pages 55 and 56.

Make sandwiches, salads and dips the night before and chill them in the refrigerator overnight.

Wash raw vegetables, cut them up and put them in individual containers so they are ready to grab and go.

If you don't have time to make a meal, fill a cooler bag with fresh fruit, juice, whole grain bread rolls or crackers, yogurt or cheese.

Keep portable meals **safe** to eat

Some foods that sit at warm temperatures in lockers, cupboards, on countertops, or out in the sun can become unsafe to eat. Foods prone to spoilage include milk products, meat, fish, eggs, as well as salads or sandwiches made with mayonnaise or salad dressing.

For safety, keep hot foods hot and cold foods cold. Invest in a thermal lined lunch bag, some small freezer packs and a good wide-mouth thermos.

Freeze plastic bottles filled with water or juice boxes to use as ice packs. You'll also benefit by having a nice cold drink to enjoy with your meal.

If you plan to heat foods later in a microwave, keep them cold in insulated bags with a freezer pack until ready to heat.

SERVES 6

Black Bean Salsa

Alice Lee
KINGSTON, ON   **P**

MAKES ABOUT 3 CUPS (750 mL)

A student at Queen's University, Alice says "this recipe is fast, easy, healthy and economical." It's also low in fat and high in fiber. Substitute 1 to 2 tsp (5 to 10 mL) dried parsley or dried basil for the fresh cilantro or parsley.

1	can (19 oz [540 mL]) black beans, rinsed and drained	1
1 cup	drained canned corn kernels	250 mL
1 cup	diced tomatoes	250 mL
1 tbsp	extra virgin olive oil	15 mL
2 tbsp	lime juice *or* cider vinegar	25 mL
2 tbsp	finely chopped fresh cilantro or parsley	25 mL
1/2 tsp	minced garlic	2 mL
1/8 tsp	black pepper	0.5 mL

TIP

For a fast meal to go, put 1/2 cup (125 mL) salsa in half a pita pocket with grated cheese and lettuce.

1. Combine all ingredients in a medium bowl and gently toss together.

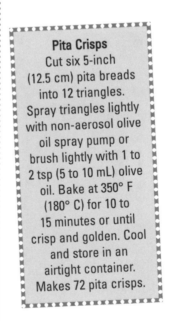

Pita Crisps
Cut six 5-inch (12.5 cm) pita breads into 12 triangles. Spray triangles lightly with non-aerosol olive oil spray pump or brush lightly with 1 to 2 tsp (5 to 10 mL) olive oil. Bake at 350° F (180° C) for 10 to 15 minutes or until crisp and golden. Cool and store in an airtight container. Makes 72 pita crisps.

Complete the meal

Serve this salsa with Pita Crisps (see recipe, at left) or baked tortilla chips, or as a condiment for any plain grilled or baked chicken, fish or meat.

Nutrition Facts

Eating more meals made with beans and corn is a great way to increase your intake of fiber and folacin.

food guide servings

GRAIN PRODUCTS	VEGETABLES & FRUIT
	1/2
	1/2
MILK PRODUCTS	MEAT & ALTERNATIVES

nutrient analysis

PER 1/2 CUP (125 ML) SERVING			
Calories	139	Carbohydrate	23.8 g
Protein	6.7 g	Dietary Fiber	5.0 g
Fat	2.9 g	Sodium	246 mg

Excellent source of folacin. **Good** source of thiamin. **High** in dietary fiber.

Fiery Verde Dip

Pamela Piotrowski, RD
Shannon Crocker, RD
HAMILTON, ON

SERVES 6

MAKES ABOUT 1 1/2 CUPS (375 mL)

This hot and spicy dip is a fresh alternative to commercially prepared guacamole and bean dips. It's low in fat and high in fiber. It goes great with pita bread triangles, Pita Crisps (see recipe, page 48), baked tortilla chips and raw veggies.

1	can (19 oz [540 mL]) white kidney or cannellini beans, rinsed and drained	1
1/2 cup	loosely packed fresh cilantro	125 mL
1/4 cup	lemon juice *or* lime juice	50 mL
1 tbsp	olive oil	15 mL
1 tsp	minced garlic	5 mL
1 or 2	jalapeño peppers, seeded and cut into chunks	1 or 2

1. In a food processor or blender, combine beans, cilantro, lemon juice, oil, garlic and peppers; blend until smooth. Chill before serving.

TIP

Cilantro – also known as fresh coriander or Chinese parsley – has a pungent flavor that you'll either love or hate. Don't confuse it with ground coriander or dried cilantro leaves which are completely different.

Nutrition Facts

Canned or dried beans, peas and lentils, as well as nuts, seeds and tahini (sesame seed paste) are all part of the "Meat & Alternatives" food group.

Make Ahead

This dip keeps in the refrigerator for up to 5 days.

Best Hummus Dip

This recipe comes from Catherine Collins in Beaconsfield, Quebec. In a blender or food processor, combine 1 can (19 oz [540 mL]) chickpeas (rinsed and drained), 2 tbsp (25 mL) tahini, 3 tbsp (45 mL) lemon juice, 1/2 tsp (2 mL) salt, 2 large cloves garlic, white part of 1 green onion and 1/4 cup (50 mL) boiling water. Blend until smooth. Stir in chopped green part of green onion; garnish with parsley. Makes 2 cups (500 mL).

Complete the meal

Spread some dip inside a whole wheat pita; fill with raw or roasted red peppers (see page 51 for technique), grated carrots and shredded lettuce. Pack in your lunch bag and treat yourself to frozen yogurt for dessert.

nutrient analysis

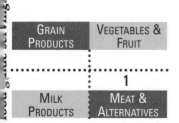

GRAIN PRODUCTS	VEGETABLES & FRUIT
	1
MILK PRODUCTS	MEAT & ALTERNATIVES

PER 1/4 CUP (50 ML) SERVING			
Calories	98	Carbohydrate	14.2 g
Protein	5.3 g	Dietary Fiber	5.5 g
Fat	2.6 g	Sodium	209 mg

Good source of folacin.
High in dietary fiber.

SERVES 5

Honey-Mustard Dip

Lorraine Fullum-Bouchard, RD
OTTAWA, ON

MAKES ABOUT 1 1/4 CUPS (300 mL)

1 cup	yogurt cheese (for technique, see page 85) *or* light sour cream	250 mL
2 tbsp	liquid honey	25 mL
2 tbsp	Dijon mustard	25 mL
3	green onions, chopped	3
1 tbsp	fresh parsley	15 mL
2 tsp	lemon juice	10 mL

1. In a food processor or blender, combine sour cream, honey, mustard, green onions, parsley and lemon juice; blend until smooth. Chill before serving.

TIP

Use this delicious dip for a sandwich spread in place of mustard or mayonnaise. It's also great as a dressing for spinach salad or coleslaw or as a sauce for cold salmon.

Nutrition Facts

Getting children to eat vegetables is often difficult – particularly at suppertime. So don't wait until the end of the day; serve vegetables as a snack after school (when kids are hungriest) and watch them disappear.

Make Ahead

This dip keeps for up to 7 days in an airtight container in the refrigerator

Herbed Yogurt Dip

Use yogurt cheese (see recipe, page 85) to whip up a quick dip. In a small bowl with an electric mixer, blend 3/4 cup (175 mL) yogurt cheese or light (5%) sour cream, 1/4 cup (50 mL) light mayonnaise, 1 tsp (5 mL) dried basil, 1/2 tsp (2 mL) minced garlic and 1/4 tsp (1 mL) granulated sugar until smooth.

Complete the meal
Put dip in a small leak-proof container and pack in an insulated lunch bag with carrot sticks, cucumber slices and a sandwich.

food guide servings

GRAIN PRODUCTS	VEGETABLES & FRUIT
1/2	
MILK PRODUCTS	MEAT & ALTERNATIVES

nutrient analysis

PER **1/4 CUP (50 mL)** SERVING			
Calories	89	Carbohydrate	13.3 g
Protein	3.8 g	Dietary Fiber	0.3 g
Fat	2.8 g	Sodium	125 mg

SERVES 6

Helen Haresign, RD
TORONTO, ON

Quick Roasted Red Pepper Dip

MAKES 1 1/2 CUPS (375 mL)

Roasted red peppers are flavorful and offer key nutrients. No wonder they are a common ingredient in many recipes. You can roast them yourself and freeze them for later use or purchase them already prepared in a jar.

Helen suggests that you can "save yourself time and money by buying a bushel (or other large amount) in late summer when they are in season. Take an evening or Saturday morning to roast them on the barbecue then freeze."

To roast peppers:
Heat barbecue (you can broil in oven as well, but it's easier and less messy on the barbecue and you can enjoy the outdoors); place several peppers on grill and cook until skins turn black. Keep turning peppers until skins are blistered and black. Place roasted peppers in large stockpot with lid. Steam will make them sweat and skin will be easier to peel off. Let peppers cool. Remove stems, seeds and skin.

Nutrition Facts
Red peppers are high in antioxidant vitamins, including beta-carotene and vitamin C.

3	roasted red bell peppers, skins and seeds removed (see technique, at left)	3
3/4 cup	feta cheese, drained and crumbled (about 6 oz [175 g])	175 mL
1/2 tsp	minced garlic	2 mL
1/4 tsp	hot pepper flakes	1 mL

1. In a food processor or blender, purée peppers, feta cheese, garlic and hot pepper flakes. Chill before serving.

Complete the meal

Serve with raw vegetables and Pita Crisps (see recipe, page 48), pita bread triangles or whole wheat crackers.

nutrient analysis

PER **1/4 CUP (50 mL)** SERVING			
Calories	58	Carbohydrate	4.6 g
Protein	2.8 g	Dietary Fiber	0.9 g
Fat	3.4 g	Sodium	175 mg

Excellent source of vitamin C. **Good** source of vitamin A, vitamin B$_{12}$.

SERVES 5

Sandy Stewart
OAKVILLE, ON

Strawberry-Apple Salsa with Cinnamon Crisps

PREHEAT OVEN TO 425° F (220° C)
LARGE NONSTICK BAKING SHEET

Fruit salsa is a refreshing snack for summer entertaining. Set the salsa out with a basket of cinnamon tortilla crisps and watch it disappear. This salsa also makes a delicious topping for vanilla-flavored yogurt or pudding.

Cinnamon Crisps

5	small (8-inch [20 cm]) flour tortillas	5
1 tbsp	granulated sugar	15 mL
1/2 tsp	cinnamon	2 mL

Strawberry-Apple Salsa

1 cup	hulled strawberries	250 mL
1	medium tart apple, peeled and diced	1
2 tbsp	liquid honey *or* brown sugar	25 mL
1/2 tsp	grated orange zest (optional)	2 mL

Nutrition Facts
Experiment with new ways to enjoy nutrient-packed fresh fruit in season. Choose different fruits each day to benefit from the variety of nutrients that each fruit provides.

1. **Cinnamon Crisps:** Brush tortillas with water; sprinkle with sugar and cinnamon. Cut into wedges. Place on baking sheet and bake for 5 minutes or until golden and crisp.

2. **Salsa:** In a medium bowl, mash strawberries; add apple, honey and, if using, orange zest. Stir to blend well. Serve with Cinnamon Crisps.

complete the meal

Enjoy with vanilla or fruit-flavored yogurt for a quick snack or as a meal to go.

food guide servings

GRAIN PRODUCTS	VEGETABLES & FRUIT
1	1/2

MILK PRODUCTS	MEAT & ALTERNATIVES

nutrient analysis

PER SERVING			
Calories	161	Carbohydrate	32.9 g
Protein	3.0 g	Dietary Fiber	2.2 g
Fat	2.4 g	Sodium	151 mg

Good source of vitamin C. **Moderate** source of dietary fiber.

SERVES 12

No-Bake Trail Mix

Marilynn Small, RD
Post Cereals
TORONTO, ON

P

MAKES 6 CUPS (1.5 L)

4 cups	Shreddies-type cereal	1 L
1 tsp	cinnamon	5 mL
1 1/2 cups	chopped mixed dried fruit	375 mL
1/2 cup	whole almonds, toasted	125 mL
1 cup	coconut (optional)	250 mL

1. Combine cereal and cinnamon in large bowl; mix in remaining ingredients.

TIP

Here's a quick and easy snack to make up and take along for a high-carbohydrate energy boost!

Prepare as needed. Keep in airtight container. Mixture will be less crisp after 1 or 2 days.

Allergy Alert

This recipe contains nuts, so check for nut allergies before serving.

Cranberry Crunchers

The next time you're craving something sweet and crunchy, yet low in fat, try one of these crunchers from Susanne Stark of Toronto, ON and Post Cereals. They're made in under 10 minutes.

Melt 1/4 cup (50 mL) butter in a large microwaveable bowl for 40 seconds. Add 1 package (8 oz [250 g]) marshmallows, tossing to coat well. Microwave on High for 1 to 1 1/2 minutes or until smooth when stirred. Stir in 1/2 tsp (2 mL) almond extract. Add in 6 cups (1.5 L) cranberry almond crunch-type cereal, stirring until coated. Press into a buttered 9- by 13-inch (22.5 by 32.5 cm) pan. Cool. Cut into squares. Makes 24 bars.

Complete the meal

Pack a container of yogurt or milk along with this trail mix for a speedy breakfast or snack to go.

food guide servings

GRAIN PRODUCTS	VEGETABLES & FRUIT
1/2	1

MILK PRODUCTS	MEAT & ALTERNATIVES

nutrient analysis

PER 1/2 CUP (125 mL) SERVING			
Calories	153	Carbohydrate	28.3 g
Protein	3.2 g	Dietary Fiber	3.2 g
Fat	3.9 g	Sodium	106 mg

Excellent source of thiamin. **Good** source of iron. **Moderate** source of dietary fiber.

Bev Callaghan, RD

SERVES 4

Egg and Mushroom Fried Rice

Ⓟ

Enjoy this as a meal or snack – it's a great way to use up leftover rice. You can easily divide the ingredients in half to serve two.

TIP
Using a small amount of highly flavored sesame oil adds great taste without adding too much fat.

Make Ahead
Serve rice for supper and pack up leftovers for lunch the next day. Keep in a cold container until ready to reheat in a microwave.

4	eggs	4
2 tsp	vegetable oil	10 mL
1 cup	sliced mushrooms	250 mL
1 tsp	minced garlic	5 mL
1 tsp	minced ginger root *or* 1/2 tsp (2 mL) ground ginger	5 mL
3 cups	cooked rice	750 mL
1/2 cup	frozen peas	125 mL
1/2 cup	chopped green onions	125 mL
1/3 cup	sodium-reduced soya sauce	75 mL
1/2 to 1 tsp	sesame oil	2 to 5 mL
1/8 tsp	black pepper	0.5 mL

1. In a small bowl, whisk eggs until well blended. Pour into a large nonstick skillet; cook undisturbed over low heat for 4 to 5 minutes or until bottom is lightly browned and mixture is almost set. Flip eggs over and cook for 1 to 2 minutes. Remove from pan; cool slightly. Cut into 1/4-inch (5 mm) strips. Set aside.

2. In the same skillet, heat oil over medium-high heat. Add mushrooms; cook for 4 to 5 minutes or until lightly browned. Add garlic and ginger; cook for 1 minute. Stir in rice, peas and onions until combined. Stir in soya sauce, sesame oil and pepper; add cooked egg strips. Cook for 2 minutes or until piping hot.

complete the meal
Finish the meal with fresh or canned fruit and frozen yogurt.

food guide servings

GRAIN PRODUCTS	VEGETABLES & FRUIT
1 1/2	1/2
	1
MILK PRODUCTS	MEAT & ALTERNATIVES

nutrient analysis

PER SERVING			
Calories	284	Carbohydrate	39.4 g
Protein	11.9 g	Dietary Fiber	2.1 g
Fat	8.3 g	Sodium	881 mg

Excellent source of niacin. **Good** source of iron, zinc, riboflavin, folacin, vitamin B$_{12}$. **Moderate** source of dietary fiber.

SERVES 1

Bev Callaghan, RD
Lynn Roblin, RD

[P]

Lunch Box Chili Rice and Beans

3-CUP (750 mL) MICROWAVE-SAFE PLASTIC CONTAINER

1 cup	cooked rice	250 mL
3/4 cup	canned kidney beans, rinsed and drained	175 mL
1/2 cup	frozen corn	125 mL
1/2 to 3/4 cup	chopped fresh tomato (about 1 medium)	125 to 175 mL
1/4 cup	diced green bell pepper	50 mL
2 tbsp	finely chopped onion	25 mL
1/4 to 1/2 tsp	chili powder	1 to 2 mL

Here's a quick, portable lunch that's low in fat and packed with fiber (an incredible 15.4 g!) and essential nutrients. It's guaranteed to perk up your lunch-time tastebuds!

The idea here is to pack up the ingredients you need for this meal the night before and, if you have access to a microwave, cook the meal at work or school. Be sure to pack this dish in an insulated lunch bag with a small ice pack.

1. In a container combine rice, beans, corn, tomato, green pepper, onion and chili powder. Stir until combined.

2. Microwave on High, loosely covered, for 2 to 3 minutes or until hot. Stir before serving.

TIP

Substitute canned diced or stewed tomatoes when fresh tomatoes are unavailable. This recipe can easily be doubled for a main meal.

Margarine and yogurt containers, plastic children's dishes and polystyrene foam containers are not appropriate for cooking and reheating in the microwave. These types of containers may release chemicals into foods when heated.

Complete the meal
With a carton of milk or a container of yogurt, you'll have a balanced meal for lunch.

nutrient analysis

GRAIN PRODUCTS	VEGETABLES & FRUIT
2	2 1/2
	1
MILK PRODUCTS	MEAT & ALTERNATIVES

PER SERVING			
Calories	447	Carbohydrate	93.9 g
Protein	18.0 g	Dietary Fiber	15.4 g
Fat	1.6 g	Sodium	429 mg

Excellent source of vitamin C, niacin, folacin. **Good** source of iron, zinc, vitamin A, thiamin, riboflavin, B_6. **Very high** in dietary fiber.

Bev Callaghan, RD
Lynn Roblin, RD

SERVES 1

P

Lunch Box Peachy Sweet Potato and Couscous

3-CUP (750 mL) MICROWAVE-SAFE PLASTIC CONTAINER

Tired of the same old sand-wiches? This tasty meal-to-go makes a delicious change of pace for the lunch-box crowd!

The idea here is to pack up the ingredients you need for this meal the night before and, if you have access to a microwave, cook the meal at work or at school.

1	small sweet potato (about 6 oz [175 g])	1
1/4 cup	uncooked couscous	50 mL
2 tbsp	raisins	25 mL
1 tsp	chicken or vegetable bouillon powder	5 mL
1/4 tsp	ground ginger	1 ml
1/8 tsp	cinnamon (optional)	0.5 mL
1	can (5 oz [142 g]) diced peaches, with juice	1
1/4 cup	water	50 mL

TIP
Use only containers labelled "microwave-safe" when cooking or reheating in the microwave. Margarine and yogurt containers, plastic children's dishes and poly-styrene foam containers are not appropriate.

1. Microwave the sweet potato on High for 2 to 2 1/2 minutes or until just cooked. Let cool; peel and dice into 1-inch (2.5 cm) pieces. Place in container.

2. Add couscous, raisins, chicken bouillon, ginger and, if using, cinnamon. Refrigerate for up to 1 day.

3. When you are ready to cook, stir in peaches and water. Microwave, loosely covered, on High for 3 minutes. Stir, cover and let stand for 2 to 3 minutes. Fluff with a fork.

Complete the meal
Pack up with a container of milk in an insulated lunch bag with a small ice pack or purchase a carton of milk. Or treat yourself to a frozen yogurt.

Variation
For a change, substitute curry powder for the ginger and cinnamon.

Add in some leftover cooked pork strips, if desired.

food guide servings

GRAIN PRODUCTS	VEGETABLES & FRUIT
1 1/2	4

MILK PRODUCTS	MEAT & ALTERNATIVES

nutrient analysis

PER SERVING			
Calories	440	Carbohydrate	100.8 g
Protein	10.4 g	Dietary Fiber	8.0 g
Fat	1.0 g	Sodium	878 mg

Excellent source of vitamin A, vitamin C, B_6, folacin. **Good** source of thiamin, riboflavin, niacin, iron. **Very high** in dietary fiber.

SERVES 8 | Barbecued Beef Satays

Lorna Driedger, RD
CALGARY, AB

MAKES 24 SATAYS

Lorna serves these satays as a main meal with rice and stir-fried vegetables. They're also great as an appetizer or snack anytime. If the weather isn't suitable for barbecuing, the satays can be broiled instead.

1 1/4 lbs	sirloin or round steak, cut into 3- by 1/2-inch (7.5 by 1 cm) strips	625 g
1/4 cup	sodium-reduced soya sauce	50 mL
1 tbsp	lemon juice	15 mL
1 tbsp	brown sugar	15 mL
1/2 tsp	minced garlic	2 mL
1/2 tsp	ground coriander	2 mL
1/4 tsp	ground cumin	1 mL
1/4 tsp	ground ginger	1 mL
	Prepared peanut sauce	

TIP

Remember to use a clean plate to bring cooked satays back in from the barbecue. Raw meat juices can contaminate cooked foods.

1. Place beef strips in a large freezer bag. Set aside.
2. In a small bowl, blend together soya sauce, lemon juice, brown sugar, garlic, coriander, cumin and ginger. Pour over beef strips; seal bag. Marinate in refrigerator for at least 4 hours or overnight.
3. Remove meat from marinade; place on small wooden skewers. Discard marinade.
4. Barbecue or broil over medium-high heat, turning once, for 4 to 5 minutes or until brown and cooked to desired doneness. Serve with your favorite peanut dipping sauce.

Make Ahead

Start marinating the beef strips the night before and the satays will only take a few minutes to prepare the next day. Soak wooden skewers for about 30 minutes to prevent them from burning on the barbecue. Be careful with skewers when young children are around.

Allergy Alert

If using peanut sauce, check for food allergies before serving.

Complete the meal

Serve as an appetizer with raw vegetables and HERBED YOGURT DIP (see recipe, page 50) or as a meal with COLESLAW FOR A CROWD (see recipe, page 82) and whole wheat rolls.

GRAIN PRODUCTS	VEGETABLES & FRUIT
	1
MILK PRODUCTS	MEAT & ALTERNATIVES

nutrient analysis

PER 3 SATAYS			
Calories	102	Carbohydrate	1.4 g
Protein	15.4 g	Dietary Fiber	0.0 g
Fat	3.5 g	Sodium	180 mg

Excellent source of vitamin B_{12}, zinc.
Good source of niacin.

SERVES 6

Shelagh Rowney
GEORGETOWN, ON

Sticky Honey-Garlic Chicken Wings

PREHEAT OVEN TO 425° F (220° C)
13- BY 9-INCH (3 L) NONSTICK BAKING PAN

Wings are a very kid-friendly meal. Shelagh likes these wings because all her children enjoy them and she gets to escape from the kitchen in record time. They're perfect for when a bunch of hungry teens hits the home front.

3 lbs	chicken wings, tips removed and split into 2 pieces at joint (about 24 pieces)	1.5 kg
1/3 cup	liquid honey	75 mL
1/4 cup	brown sugar	50 mL
3 tbsp	soya sauce	45 mL
2 tbsp	lemon juice *or* vinegar	25 mL
1 tsp	garlic powder	5 mL
1/2 tsp	ground ginger, optional	2 mL

TIP

This is a very quick recipe to prepare but the wings do take time to cook – so plan accordingly. You can save time with pre-separated chicken wings (wing tips removed) available at some grocery stores. Chicken drumettes can also be substituted for all or half of the chicken wings.

Make Ahead

Wings can be made ahead and refrigerated for up to 2 days or frozen (thaw before reheating). Reheat in a single layer on baking sheet for 10 to 15 minutes at 350° F (180° C).

1. Place wings in a single layer in baking pan. Bake in preheated oven for 20 minutes; drain fat.

2. Meanwhile, in a bowl, blend together honey, brown sugar, soya sauce, lemon juice, garlic powder and, if using, ginger. Set aside.

3. Pour sauce over wings. Reduce oven temperature to 400° F (200° C); bake, turning twice during cooking time, for 40 to 45 minutes or until wings are browned and glazed.

complete the meal
Serve with rice and MANDARIN ORANGE SALAD (see recipe, page 89) or any fresh, frozen or canned vegetable. For a snack, serve with raw vegetable. and HONEY MUSTARD DIP (see recipe, page 50) and whole-grain rolls.

food guide servings

GRAIN PRODUCTS	VEGETABLES & FRUIT
	1
MILK PRODUCTS	MEAT & ALTERNATIVES

nutrient analysis

PER SERVING (4 WINGS)			
Calories	307	Carbohydrate	25.6 g
Protein	20 g	Dietary Fiber	0.2 g
Fat	14.1 g	Sodium	578 mg

Excellent source of niacin. **Good** source of zinc, vitamin B$_6$.

MAKES 10

Curried Chicken Salad Wraps

Cheryl Wren
TORONTO, ON   [P]

Stuff this chicken mixture into mini pita breads for a tasty appetizer. It also makes a great sandwich filling for pumpernickel bread!

TIP

If you don't have any cooked chicken on hand, pick up a cooked chicken at the grocery store. One cooked deli chicken yields about 3 cups (750 mL) cubed cooked chicken. Cooked turkey can be substituted for the chicken.

Nutrition Facts

To cut back on fat, substitute 1/3 cup (75 mL) yogurt or light sour cream for half of the light mayonnaise.

Allergy Alert

This recipe contains almonds, which can easily be omitted if someone you are serving has a nut allergy.

3 cups	cubed cooked chicken	750 mL
1 cup	chopped celery	250 mL
1 cup	halved seedless red or green grapes	250 mL
1/2 cup	toasted slivered almonds (see technique, page 124)	125 mL
1 tbsp	lemon juice	15 mL
3/4 tsp	curry powder	4 mL
2/3 cup	light mayonnaise	150 mL
	Salt and black pepper to taste	
10	large (10-inch [25 cm]) flour tortillas	10
10	lettuce leaves	10

1. In a large bowl, stir together chicken, celery, grapes, almonds, lemon juice, curry powder, mayonnaise and salt and pepper to taste.

2. Place one lettuce leaf on each tortilla. Divide chicken mixture evenly down the center of each lettuce leaf. Fold up bottom and roll up tortilla.

Complete the meal
Serve these wraps with CHILLED MELON AND MANGO SOUP *(see recipe, page 72.)*

GRAIN PRODUCTS	VEGETABLES & FRUIT
2	1/2
	1
MILK PRODUCTS	MEAT & ALTERNATIVES

nutrient analysis

PER WRAP			
Calories	366	Carbohydrate	37.9 g
Protein	18.8 g	Dietary Fiber	2.8 g
Fat	15.4 g	Sodium	425 mg

Excellent source of thiamin, niacin. **Good** source of iron, zinc, riboflavin, vitamin B_6. **Moderate** source of fiber.

MAKES 10 Favorite Chicken Fajitas

Cindy Felix
BRAMPTON, ON

Cindy invented this recipe out of necessity, since her husband Bruce has little taste for vegetables. She says she is always looking for new ways to work them into his diet. This recipe is delicious — her husband is a lucky guy!

TIP

Serve this dish with a variety of toppings such as shredded lettuce, diced tomatoes, chopped green onions, grated cheese and sour cream and let family members assemble their own fajitas.

Nutrition Facts

Buying poultry with bones and skin already removed speeds up preparation time and helps you cut back on fat.

Complete the meal

Finish the meal with a serving of lime-flavored yogurt or sherbet.

1 lb	boneless skinless chicken breasts, cut into strips	500 g
2 tbsp	balsamic vinegar	25 mL
1 tbsp	soya sauce	15 mL
1 tbsp	Russian-style salad dressing	15 mL
1/2 tsp	garlic powder	2 mL
1/2 tsp	crushed red chili peppers (optional)	2 mL
1 tbsp	vegetable oil	15 mL
1 cup	sliced green bell pepper, cut into 2-inch (5 cm) strips	250 mL
1 cup	sliced red bell pepper, cut into 2-inch (5 cm) strips	250 mL
1 cup	zucchini, cut into 2-inch (5 cm) strips	250 mL
1 cup	sliced mushrooms	250 mL
1/2 cup	sliced onions	125 mL
10	large (10-inch [25 cm]) flour tortillas	10

1. In a medium bowl, stir together chicken, vinegar, soya sauce, salad dressing, garlic powder and, if using, red chili peppers; blend well. Set aside.

2. In a large nonstick skillet, heat oil over medium-high heat. Add green pepper, red pepper, zucchini, mushrooms and onions; cook for 4 to 5 minutes. Add chicken mixture; cook for 5 to 6 minutes or until chicken is no longer pink in the center.

3. Warm tortillas in oven. Divide mixture evenly amongst tortillas. Add toppings (see Tip, at left) as desired. Roll up tortillas. Serve hot.

food guide servings

GRAIN PRODUCTS	VEGETABLES & FRUIT
2	1/2
	1/2
MILK PRODUCTS	MEAT & ALTERNATIVES

nutrient analysis

PER FAJITA			
Calories	270	Carbohydrate	35.4 g
Protein	15.8 g	Dietary Fiber	2.5 g
Fat	6.9 g	Sodium	413 mg

Excellent source of thiamin, niacin, vitamin B_6. **Good** source of iron, vitamin C. **Moderate** source of dietary fiber.

MAKES 10

Hurry-Up Fill-Me-Up Burritos

Susan Blanchard
ROTHESAY, NB   P

Susan says these are popular after-school snacks for her ever-starving teenage boys – and easy enough that the boys can make the burritos themselves. They're ready in 5 minutes from start to finish. Add sour cream, shredded lettuce and extra salsa, if desired.

1 cup	cooked rice	250 mL
1	can (14 oz [398 mL]) kidney beans, rinsed and drained	1
1 cup	corn kernels, canned or frozen	250 mL
3/4 cup	prepared salsa	175 mL
10	large (10-inch [25 cm]) flour tortillas, warmed	10
1 1/4 cups	shredded Cheddar cheese	300 mL

Food Fast

Use pre-packaged shredded cheese and leftover rice.

These burritos can also be prepared in the microwave: In a bowl stir together rice, beans, corn and salsa. Divide mixture between tortillas; sprinkle with cheese. Roll up. Microwave for 30 to 40 seconds or until heated through.

Nutrition Facts

Encouraging teens to eat more bean-based meals is a great way to increase their fiber intake.

Variation

Substitute black beans or white kidney beans for the red kidney beans.

1. In a nonstick pan over medium heat, stir together rice, beans, corn and salsa. Cook for 3 to 4 minutes or until warmed through.

2. Divide mixture evenly between tortillas. Sprinkle with cheese. Roll up tortillas.

complete the meal
Enjoy with crunchy raw vegetables or a piece of fruit and a glass of milk.

food guide servings

GRAIN PRODUCTS	VEGETABLES & FRUIT
2	1/2
1/4	1/4
MILK PRODUCTS	MEAT & ALTERNATIVES

nutrient analysis

PER BURRITO			
Calories	318	Carbohydrate	47.5 g
Protein	12.0 g	Dietary Fiber	4.9 g
Fat	9.0 g	Sodium	502 mg

Excellent source of thiamin. **Good** source of iron, riboflavin, niacin. **High** in dietary fiber.

SERVES 2

Bev Callaghan, RD

Swiss Chard Frittata in a Pita

This dish makes a delicious quick meal or snack. If you don't have any pita bread on hand, serve with whole grain toast.

TIP

Chopped fresh spinach can easily be substituted for the Swiss chard. Experiment with other greens, too, such as collard greens, kale, mustard greens, dandelion greens and rapini. They're all great substitutes for the chard in this recipe.

Nutrition Facts

While this dish is already a good source of fiber, you can get even more fiber by using whole-wheat pita bread instead of white pita bread.

Complete the meal

Serve with Salsa Fresca (see recipe, page 42), prepared salsa or, if desired, sliced fresh tomato.

4	eggs	4
1 tbsp	water	15 mL
1 tsp	olive oil	5 mL
1/4 cup	chopped onions	50 mL
1/2 tsp	minced garlic	2 mL
2 cups	packed chopped Swiss chard	500 mL
2 tbsp	chopped fresh basil (or 1/2 tsp [2 mL] dried)	25 mL
1/4 cup	grated Parmesan cheese	50 mL
2	small 6-inch (15 cm) pita breads	2

1. In a small bowl, whisk together eggs and water. Set aside.

2. In a small 8-inch (20 cm) nonstick skillet, heat oil over medium-high heat. Add onions and garlic; cook for 1 to 2 minutes. Stir in chard and basil (it will cook down; if necessary, add it in 2 batches); cook for 3 to 4 minutes or until chard is wilted. Remove from pan; set aside.

3. Wipe skillet and place over medium heat. Add half the chard mixture and half the egg mixture. Cook for 3 to 5 minutes or until browned on the bottom with some of the top still not set; sprinkle with cheese. Flip frittata over; cook for 1 to 2 minutes or until browned and completely set. Remove from pan and cut in half. Repeat procedure with remaining ingredients to make second frittata.

4. Cut pitas in half; place frittata halves inside each half.

food guide servings

Grain Products	Vegetables & Fruit
2	2
1/2	1
Milk Products	Meat & Alternatives

nutrient analysis

PER SERVING			
Calories	431	Carbohydrate	43.2 g
Protein	26.7 g	Dietary Fiber	4.0 g
Fat	16.9 g	Sodium	849 mg

Excellent source of calcium, iron, zinc, vitamin A, vitamin C, riboflavin, niacin, folacin, vitamin B_{12}. **Good** source of thiamin, vitamin B_6. **High** in dietary fiber.

SERVES 8

Tuna Salad Melt

Bev Callaghan, RD   P

Older children and teens can make these easily in a toaster oven. The tuna mixture also makes a great filling for sandwiches, wraps, pita bread, and for serving on top of salad greens or spinach. You can substitute salmon for the tuna.

Nutrition Facts

One way to cut back on fat in tuna or egg salads is to use yogurt or yogurt cheese (see page 85) as a substitute for some of the mayonnaise.

2	cans (6 oz [170 g]) water-packed tuna, drained	2
1/4 cup	finely chopped celery	50 mL
1/4 cup	finely chopped sweet pickle *or* sweet relish	50 mL
1/4 cup	finely chopped red or green bell pepper (optional)	50 mL
1/4 cup	light mayonnaise	50 mL
2 tbsp	low-fat plain yogurt	25 mL
1 tbsp	lemon juice *or* pickle juice	15 mL
1	French stick or baguette	1
1/2 cup	grated Cheddar cheese	125 mL

1. In a bowl stir together tuna, celery, pickle, red pepper, mayonnaise, yogurt and lemon juice. Blend well.

2. Slice French stick in half lengthwise. Cut each half into 4 equal portions, making 8 pieces; place on baking sheet. Toast under broiler for 1 to 2 minutes or until golden. Remove from broiler; spread tuna mixture evenly over each piece. Sprinkle with cheese. Broil for 2 to 3 minutes or until cheese is melted and golden.

complete the meal

Serve with sliced cantaloupe, a glass of milk and LUSCIOUS LEMON BARS (see recipe, page 165).

Variation

Tuna salad wrap: Fill flour tortillas with tuna mixture and grated cheese. Fold up and serve cold or microwave on High for 30 to 45 seconds or until cheese is melted. For a cold salad wrap, be adventurous and try adding any shredded vegetable such as purple cabbage, grated carrots, zucchini, arugula, mustard greens, kale or spinach.

nutrient analysis

GRAIN PRODUCTS	VEGETABLES & FRUIT
1	
	1/2
MILK PRODUCTS	MEAT & ALTERNATIVES

PER SERVING			
Calories	208	Carbohydrate	23.6 g
Protein	14.0 g	Dietary Fiber	0.6 g
Fat	6.1 g	Sodium	477 mg

Excellent source of niacin, vitamin B_{12}.

SERVES 4

Lynn Roblin, RD

Red Pepper and Goat Cheese Pizza

Here's a fast and tasty treat that makes a great change from the standard pepperoni pizza. Served warm or cold, it's terrific for lunch or a light supper — or even breakfast!

TIP

Pizza typically contains a significant amount of fat. To reduce your fat intake, try your next pizza with more vegetable toppings — and fewer high-fat toppings such as pepperoni, sausage, bacon and olives.

Food Fast

Microwave 2 slices of pizza on High for 1 minute. Wrap in foil and put in an insulated lunch bag. Add a piece of fruit and a pudding for a balanced meal.

PREHEAT OVEN TO 400° F (200° C) IF USING FLATBREAD
OR 450° F (230° C) IF USING PIZZA DOUGH
PIZZA PAN OR BAKING SHEET

1	12-inch (30 cm) round flatbread *or* enough pizza dough for a 12-inch (30 cm) pizza	1
1 tbsp	olive oil	15 mL
1 cup	grated mozzarella cheese	250 mL
1/4 cup	crumbled goat cheese	50 mL
1	large red bell pepper, thinly sliced	1
1	large tomato, sliced	1
1/4 cup	sliced black olives	50 mL
1/4 cup	sweet Vidalia onion, sliced (optional)	50 mL
1 tsp	dried basil (or 2 tbsp [25 mL] chopped fresh basil)	5 mL

1. Place flatbread on baking sheet. Alternatively, if using pizza dough, spread out dough on lightly greased pizza pan to make a 12-inch (30 cm) circle.

2. Brush olive oil on top of flatbread or pizza dough. Sprinkle with mozzarella cheese. Top with goat cheese, red pepper, tomato, black olives, onion and basil.

3. Bake pizza in the bottom half of preheated oven for 10 to 15 minutes or until crust is golden and filling is bubbly.

complete the meal

Serve with bagged ready-to-eat tossed green salad and a low-fat bottled salad dressing.

food guide servings

GRAIN PRODUCTS	VEGETABLES & FRUIT
2	1
3/4	
MILK PRODUCTS	MEAT & ALTERNATIVES

nutrient analysis

PER SERVING			
Calories	373	Carbohydrate	39.8 g
Protein	14.1 g	Dietary Fiber	2.6 g
Fat	17.7 g	Sodium	585 mg

Excellent source of vitamin C, vitamin A. **Good** source of calcium, iron, thiamin, riboflavin, niacin, folacin. **Moderate** source of dietary fiber.

SOUTHWESTERN SWEET POTATO SOUP (PAGE 75) ➤
OVERLEAF: LUNCH BOX CHILI RICE AND BEANS (PAGE 55) • NO-BAKE TRAIL MIX (PAGE 53)

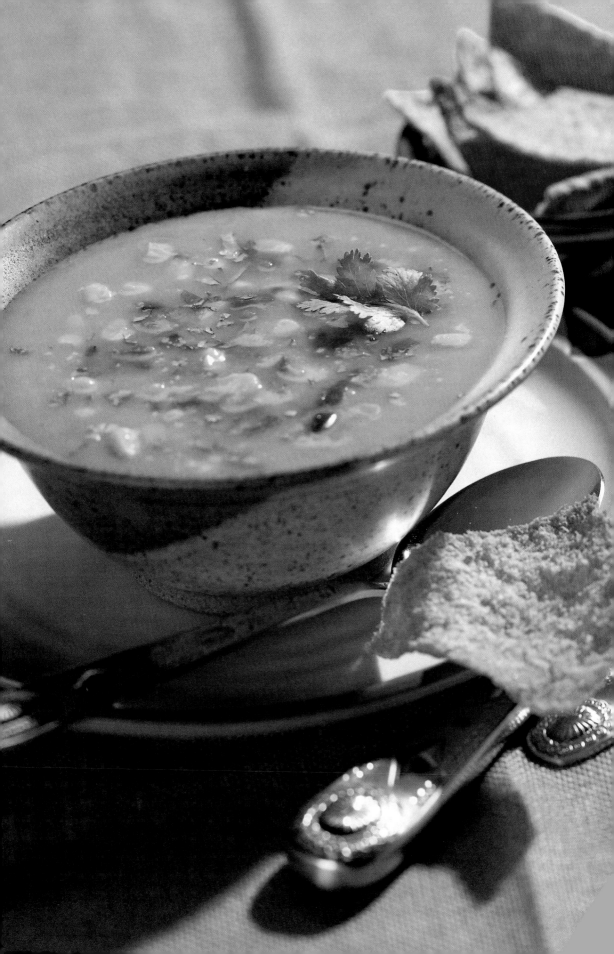

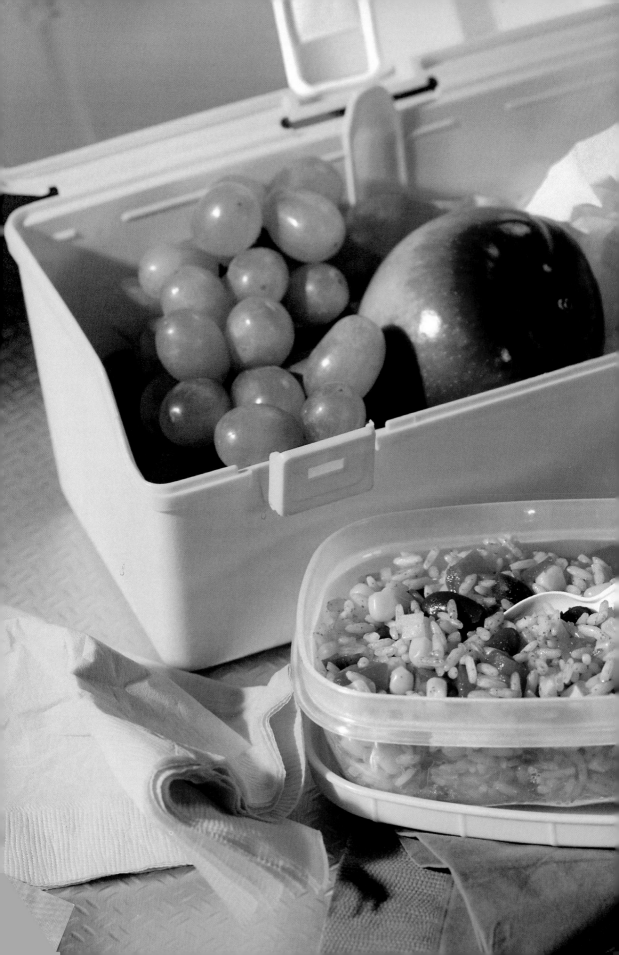

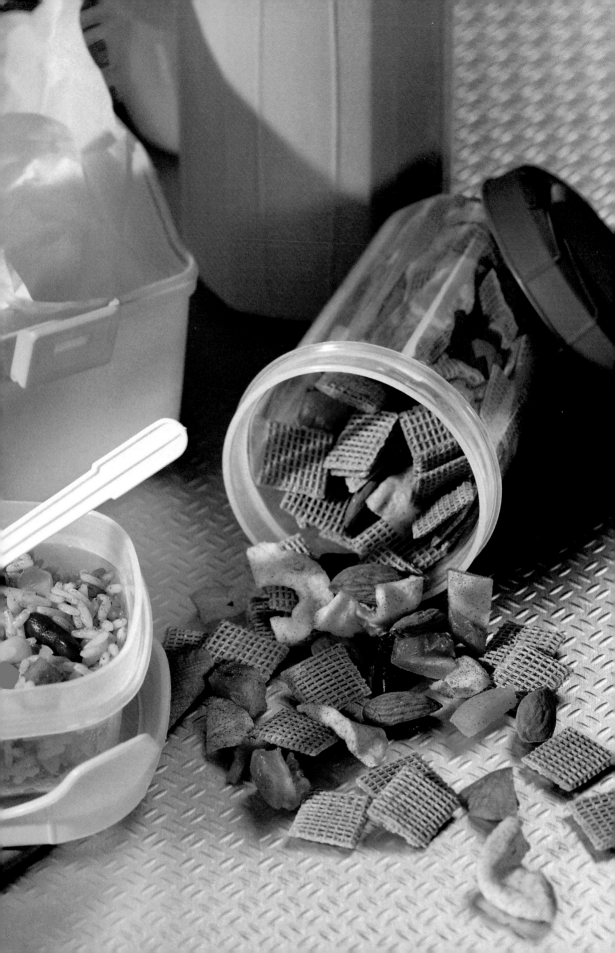

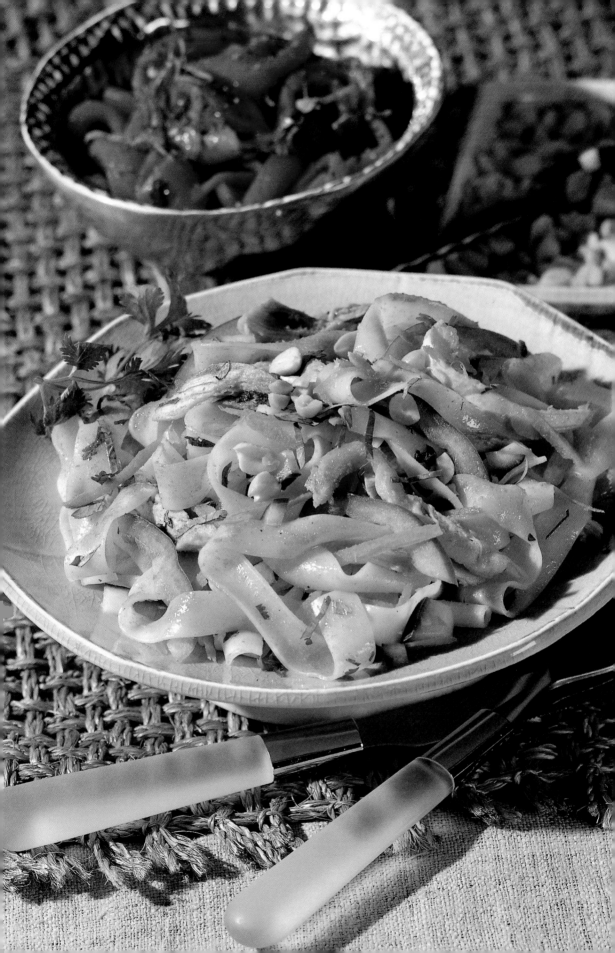

SUPER SOUPS

◄ VIETNAMESE CHICKEN AND RICE NOODLE SALAD (PAGE 94)

Here you'll find great recipes that include soups you stir up quickly and eat right away, as well as soups that you can make ahead and store in your refrigerator or freezer until needed. These soups are all easy to make, and quick and delicious to eat.

Fast and easy nutrition in a BOWL

A pot of soup kept warm on the stove makes a ready meal for family members as they pass through the kitchen at different times. Soup is also a transportable meal that can be popped into a thermos and eaten at work or at school.

Soups are a practical way to use up leftover cooked vegetables, meat or poultry.

Adding beans or lentils will boost your fiber intake and make your soup more satisfying.

Making SOUP part of a balanced meal

While soups can be meals by themselves, they can also add variety and extra nutrients as part of a more substantial meal. When soup is the main component of a meal, balance it with foods from each of the four food groups.

Each recipe features balanced meal suggestions. Here are a few more soup combinations you can try.

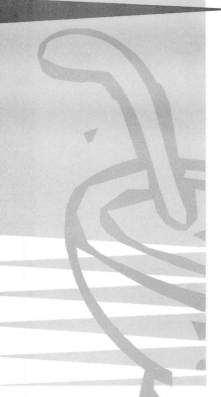

Lentil soup
with wheat crackers and
cheese, carrots and dip.

. . . .

Puréed vegetable soup
with a bagel and melted
Cheddar cheese.

. . . .

Minestrone soup with a
tuna sandwich and yogurt.

. . . .

Tomato soup with hummus
on pita bread and milk.

. . . .

The wonderful thing about soup is that you can make it from just about anything. The Great Food Fast Pantry List (pages 11 to 12) includes many possible ingredients, such as canned beans and tomatoes, fresh or frozen vegetables, noodles, rice or couscous, dried herbs, as well as soup bases like bouillon cubes or canned broth. So go ahead – be adventurous. The possibilities are endless.

give a **nutrient** **boost** to soups

Cheese soup
Make with milk and add puréed cooked broccoli or cauliflower. For extra spice, add a dash of hot pepper sauce.

Chicken broth
Whisk an egg into the soup when hot.

Chicken noodle or chicken with rice soup
Add frozen mixed vegetables or leftover cooked vegetables.

Mushroom or celery soup
Make with milk and mix in diced cooked potatoes, corn kernels and canned baby clams for a satisfying clam chowder.

Tomato soup
Make with milk to increase calcium and stir in chopped fresh tomatoes and basil. Add grated Cheddar cheese for even more calcium.

Vegetable soup
Add cooked meat or poultry.

Vegetable or noodle soups
Add some canned or cooked kidney beans, black beans, navy beans or lentils.

Watch those salty soups

Some people, particularly those with high blood pressure, need to be careful about their sodium intake – particularly with commercially prepared soups, which often contain large amounts of salt.

Powdered soup mixes, bouillon cubes, canned soups and broths are all relatively high in salt. Many of these products also contain monosodium glutamate (MSG), which adds even more sodium.

If you are concerned about salt, check food labels, as well as the sodium values listed for each recipe.

SERVES 6

Joanne Saunders
SURREY, BC [P]

Asian Turkey and Noodle Soup

MAKES 6 CUPS (1.5 L)

This soup tastes great made with fresh turkey breast, but you can also use leftover cooked turkey (about 1 cup [250 mL]). If using cooked turkey, skip the stir-fry step and add the turkey with the broth in Step 1.

TIP

Sesame oil is made from roasted sesame seeds and is used for flavoring many Asian dishes. The darker the oil, the more intense the flavor. A little goes a long way, so add it sparingly. Keep refrigerated after opening.

Grated ginger root and chopped garlic are sold preserved in jars at most supermarkets. While not as flavorful as fresh, they are great time savers.

Nutrition Facts

If you are concerned about sodium, use light soya sauce instead of the regular variety. One tbsp (15 mL) regular soya sauce contains 1037 mg sodium; the same amount of sodium-reduced or light soya sauce contains only 605 mg.

2 tsp	vegetable oil	10 mL
8 oz	boneless skinless turkey breast, cut into strips	250 g
1 cup	sliced mushrooms	250 mL
2	cans (each 10 oz [284 mL]) chicken broth	2
3 cups	water	750 mL
1 tsp	minced garlic	5 mL
1 tsp	grated ginger root	5 mL
1 tbsp	rice wine vinegar *or* lemon juice	15 mL
1 tbsp	soya sauce	15 mL
1 tsp	sesame oil	5 mL
1/4 tsp	hot pepper sauce	1 mL
4 oz	fresh chow mein *or* rice noodles	125 g
1 1/2 cups	snow peas, trimmed and cut into 1-inch (2.5 cm) pieces	375 mL
1/2 cup	chopped green onions	125 mL

1. In a large saucepan, heat oil over medium-high heat. Add turkey and stir-fry for 2 to 3 minutes. Add mushrooms; cook for 2 to 3 minutes. Add broth, water, garlic and ginger; bring to a boil. Add vinegar, soya sauce, sesame oil, hot pepper sauce and noodles; reduce heat and simmer for 3 to 4 minutes.

2. Add snow peas and green onions; simmer for 1 to 2 minutes. Serve immediately.

complete the meal

Serve as an elegant first course when entertaining or have with a sandwich and a glass of milk.

food guide servings

GRAIN PRODUCTS	VEGETABLES & FRUIT
1/2	1/2
	1/2
MILK PRODUCTS	MEAT & ALTERNATIVES

nutrient analysis

PER SERVING			
Calories	165	Carbohydrate	14.1 g
Protein	16.6 g	Dietary Fiber	1.4 g
Fat	4.4 g	Sodium	837 mg

Excellent source of niacin. **Good** source of folacin, vitamin B_{12}.

SERVES 8

Fleur-Ange Joubert
ANCIENNE LORETTE, PQ
P

Beef, Vegetable and Bean Soup

MAKES 9 CUPS (2.25 L)

12 oz	lean ground beef	375 g
2 tsp	minced garlic	10 mL
1/2 cup	chopped onions	125 mL
1 cup	chopped carrots	250 mL
1 cup	chopped celery or fennel	250 mL
1 cup	chopped zucchini	250 mL
1 tsp	dried basil	5 mL
1	bay leaf	1
6 cups	beef stock	1.5 L
1	can (28 oz [796 mL]) whole tomatoes	1
1/2 cup	macaroni (or any other small pasta)	125 mL
3 cups	fresh chopped spinach	750 mL
1	can (19 oz [540 mL]) mixed beans, rinsed and drained	1

1. In a large saucepan or Dutch oven, brown beef over medium-high heat. Add garlic, onions, carrots, celery and zucchini; cook for 5 minutes. Add basil, bay leaf, stock and tomatoes; bring to a boil. Reduce heat and simmer, covered, for 10 minutes.

2. Add pasta; cook for another 5 to 6 minutes. Add spinach and beans; cook for another 3 to 4 minutes. Remove bay leaf before serving.

Complete the meal
Enjoy this soup accompanied by a bagel topped with melted Cheddar cheese.

TIP

If you don't have beef stock, substitute two cans (each 10 oz [284 mL]) beef broth plus 3 1/2 cups (875 mL) water or substitute 6 beef bouillon cubes or sachets (2 tbsp [25 mL]) plus 6 cups (1.5 L) water.

Any 19-oz (540 mL) can of beans can be used in place of the mixed beans. Try kidney, romano or white pea beans.

If you don't have any zucchini, substitute an equal amount of frozen peas, green beans or corn.

Nutrition Facts

This soup is very high in fiber and is packed with many essential nutrients, including folacin. It's a great choice for women who are trying to add more iron and folic acid to their meals.

Make Ahead

This soup keeps for up to 3 days in the refrigerator or 4 months in the freezer.

food guide servings

GRAIN PRODUCTS	VEGETABLES & FRUIT
	2
	1
MILK PRODUCTS	MEAT & ALTERNATIVES

nutrient analysis

PER SERVING			
Calories	225	Carbohydrate	23.7 g
Protein	16.7 g	Dietary Fiber	6.8 g
Fat	7.5 g	Sodium	967 mg

Excellent source of zinc, vitamin A, niacin, folacin, vitamin B_{12}. **Good** source of iron, riboflavin, vitamin B_6. **Very high** in dietary fiber.

SERVES 6

Patricia Mialkowsky
SASKATOON, SK [P]

Caribbean Ham and Black Bean Soup

MAKES 7 CUPS (1.75 L)

Here's a very simple soup that's low in fat and high in fiber. It's also an excellent source of folacin.

Food Fast
This makes a nice hot meal-to-go. Heat it up in the morning, pop into a thermos and enjoy it with your lunch.

Make Ahead
This soup can be made ahead and kept up to 3 days in the refrigerator or frozen for up to 4 months. If you are using leftover ham, be sure that it's not more than a day or two old.

1/2 cup	chopped onions	125 mL
3 cups	water	750 mL
1	can (19 oz [540 mL]) black beans, rinsed and drained	1
1	can (19 oz [540 mL]) stewed tomatoes	1
1 cup	diced cooked ham	250 mL
1/2 cup	frozen corn kernels	125 mL
1/4 cup	long grain rice	50 mL
1 tbsp	lime juice	15 mL
2 tsp	brown sugar	10 mL
1 tsp	hot pepper sauce	5 mL
1/2 tsp	ground cumin	2 mL
1/4 tsp	ground ginger	1 mL

1. In a large saucepan sprayed with vegetable spray, cook onions over medium-high heat for 3 to 4 minutes or until tender. Stir in water, beans, tomatoes, ham, corn, rice, lime juice, brown sugar, hot pepper sauce, cumin and ginger; bring to a boil. Reduce heat and simmer, covered, for 15 to 20 minutes or until rice is tender.

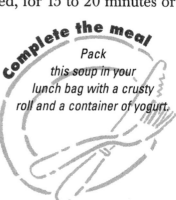

Complete the meal
Pack this soup in your lunch bag with a crusty roll and a container of yogurt.

food guide servings

GRAIN PRODUCTS	VEGETABLES & FRUIT
	1
	1
MILK PRODUCTS	MEAT & ALTERNATIVES

nutrient analysis

PER SERVING			
Calories	191	Carbohydrate	32.9 g
Protein	12.5 g	Dietary Fiber	5.4 g
Fat	1.9 g	Sodium	683 mg

Excellent source of thiamin, folacin. **Good** source of iron, zinc, niacin. **High** in dietary fiber.

SERVES 6

Carrot-Orange Soup

Mary Persi
TORONTO, ON

P

MAKES 7 CUPS (1.75 L)

Oranges and carrots make a delicious flavor combination. Enjoy this soup at home or heat it up and add to your lunch bag for a healthy hot treat.

2 tbsp	butter *or* margarine	25 mL
1/2 cup	chopped onions	125 mL
4 cups	sliced carrots	1 L
4 cups	chicken stock *or* vegetable stock	1 L
1/2 cup	orange juice	125 mL
1/2 tsp	ground nutmeg	2 mL
1/4 tsp	ground white pepper	1 mL
1 cup	milk	250 mL

TIP

To make a creamier soup, use evaporated milk.

1. In a large saucepan, heat butter over medium-high heat. Add onions and cook for 4 to 5 minutes or until softened. Add carrots and stock; bring to a boil. Reduce heat and simmer for 15 to 20 minutes or until carrots are very soft. Stir in orange juice, nutmeg and pepper.

2. In a food processor or blender, purée carrot mixture in batches until smooth.

3. Return soup to pan; stir in milk. Simmer over very low heat for 2 to 3 minutes or until heated through.

Nutrition Facts

Including soup as a meal or part of a meal is a simple way for younger and older folks to get more nutrient-rich vegetables into their day.

Complete the meal

Enjoy this soup with a TUNA SALAD MELT (see recipe, page 63) or a sandwich. Have pudding for dessert.

Make Ahead

Prepare a double batch of this soup. After Step 2, pour half the soup into a container with a tight-fitting lid. Freeze for up to 3 to 4 months. When ready to enjoy, defrost, add milk and heat through.

food guide servings

GRAIN PRODUCTS	VEGETABLES & FRUIT
	1 1/2

MILK PRODUCTS	MEAT & ALTERNATIVES

nutrient analysis

PER SERVING			
Calories	130	Carbohydrate	13.9 g
Protein	5.8 g	Dietary Fiber	2.3 g
Fat	5.8 g	Sodium	628 mg

Excellent source of vitamin A. **Good** source of niacin. **Moderate** source of dietary fiber.

SERVES 4

Bev Callaghan, RD Ⓟ

Chilled Melon and Mango Soup

MAKES ABOUT 3 1/2 CUPS (875 mL)

2 cups	cubed cantaloupe	500 mL
1 cup	diced mango	250 mL
3/4 cup	orange juice	175 mL
1/2 cup	lower-fat plain yogurt	125 mL
2 tbsp	lime juice	25 mL
2 tbsp	liquid honey	25 mL
	Chopped fresh mint (optional)	

TIP

This delicious, rich-tasting soup is perfect for a hot summer day. It can be the main dish in a fast and elegant lunch or poured into a tall glass for a nutrient-packed antioxidant cocktail. You can also put the soup into a thermos for a meal-to-go.

Nutrition Facts

Mangoes are rich in flavor and high in beta-carotene. They are ready to eat when their skins have turned yellow-orange or red in color and are soft to the touch.

Make Ahead

This soup can be refrigerated for up to 3 days but does not freeze well.

1. In a food processor or blender, combine cantaloupe and mango; purée until smooth. Add orange juice, yogurt, lime juice and honey. Blend until combined.

2. Chill before serving. Serve sprinkled with mint, if desired.

Complete the meal

Enjoy this soup with CURRIED CHICKEN SALAD WRAPS (see recipe, page 59) for a special lunch.

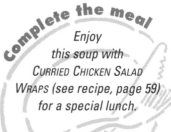

food guide servings

GRAIN PRODUCTS	VEGETABLES & FRUIT
	2
MILK PRODUCTS	MEAT & ALTERNATIVES

nutrient analysis

PER SERVING			
Calories	131	Carbohydrate	30.4 g
Protein	2.9 g	Dietary Fiber	1.6 g
Fat	1.0 g	Sodium	30 mg

Excellent source of vitamin C, vitamin A. **Good** source of folacin.

SERVES 6

Lynn Roblin, RD P

Chunky Vegetable Lentil Soup

MAKES 6 CUPS (1.5 L)

2 cups	water	500 mL
1	vegetable bouillon cube	1
1 cup	chopped carrots	250 mL
1	can (28 oz [796 mL]) diced tomatoes	1
1	can (19 oz [540 mL]) lentils, rinsed and drained	1
2 tsp	minced garlic	10 mL
1 tsp	dried basil	5 mL
1/2 tsp	ground thyme	2 mL
1/2 tsp	cumin	2 mL

TIP

This super-speedy soup will warm you up on a cold day. The cumin gives it a nice flavor that's similar to chili. This soup is very easy for older children or teens to make, so leave the recipe out and encourage whoever gets home first to get supper started.

Nutrition Facts

Lentils come in many colors but the most common are red, brown and green. They are available in cans, which makes them easy to add to soups, stews and casseroles. They can also be added cold to salads.

1. In a large saucepan, bring water to a boil. Add vegetable bouillon cube; stir until dissolved.

2. Add carrots; reduce heat to medium and cook, covered, for 10 minutes.

3. Add tomatoes, lentils, garlic, basil, thyme and cumin; reduce heat to medium-low and cook, stirring often, for 10 minutes or until carrots are tender.

Complete the meal

Serve with warm crusty bread and cheese.

Food Fast

Heat soup in the microwave, pour into a thermos and pack into a lunch bag with a sandwich and a piece of fruit. All you need to balance your meal is a container of milk.

food guide servings

GRAIN PRODUCTS	VEGETABLES & FRUIT
	1 1/2
	1/2
MILK PRODUCTS	MEAT & ALTERNATIVES

nutrient analysis

PER SERVING			
Calories	118	Carbohydrate	22.1 g
Protein	7.7 g	Dietary Fiber	4.8 g
Fat	0.7 g	Sodium	541 mg

Excellent source of vitamin A, folacin. **Good** source of iron, vitamin B$_6$. **High** in dietary fiber.

SERVES 8

Seafood Chowder

Seanna Callaghan
TORONTO, ON

MAKES 8 CUPS (2 L)

2 cups	diced potatoes	500 mL
1 cup	diced carrots	250 mL
1/2 cup	chopped onions	125 mL
2	cans (each 14 oz [398 mL]) evaporated 2% milk	2
1 cup	frozen peas	250 mL
1	can (5 oz [142 g]) clams, drained	1
1 cup	chopped cooked shrimp	250 mL
1 cup	chopped cooked crab or any type of cooked fish fillets	250 mL
1/2 tsp	salt	2 mL
	Black pepper	
1/2 cup	finely chopped green onions or chives	125 mL
	Paprika	
1 cup	seasoned croutons	250 mL

TIP

Substitute any combination of cooked seafood that you prefer for the clams, shrimp and crab. Just make sure that the total amount of seafood is about 3 cups (750 mL).

Nutrition Facts

Evaporated milk gives a creamy texture to soups without adding a lot of extra fat. It can be used in place of cream in many recipes.

Make Ahead

Prepare soup through Step 2 up to 2 days ahead and store in refrigerator. This soup does not freeze well.

1. Place potatoes, carrots and onions in a large saucepan. Add just enough water to cover, about 2 cups (500 mL); bring to a boil. Reduce heat and simmer, uncovered, for 10 to 12 minutes or until tender.

2. Add milk and peas; simmer for 4 to 5 minutes. Add clams, shrimp and crab; simmer for 2 to 3 minutes or until heated through. Season with salt and pepper to taste.

3. Serve garnished with onions, paprika and croutons.

complete the meal

Serve with whole grain bread or rolls.

food guide servings

GRAIN PRODUCTS	VEGETABLES & FRUIT
	1
1	1
MILK PRODUCTS	MEAT & ALTERNATIVES

nutrient analysis

PER SERVING			
Calories	225	Carbohydrate	26.1 g
Protein	21.1 g	Dietary Fiber	2.1 g
Fat	3.9 g	Sodium	532 mg

Excellent source of vitamin A, riboflavin, niacin, vitamin B_{12}, calcium, iron. **Good** source of vitamin C, folacin, zinc. **Moderate** source of dietary fiber.

SERVES 6

Southwestern Sweet Potato Soup

Claudette Turnbull, RD
ST. CATHARINES, ON

MAKES 6 CUPS (1.5 L)

Nutrition Facts

Eating more dark-orange and red vegetables – such as sweet potatoes and red peppers – helps increase your intake of beta-carotene (the plant form of vitamin A), vitamin C and other antioxidants.

1 tbsp	olive oil	15 mL
1/2 cup	chopped onions	125 mL
2 cups	diced peeled sweet potatoes	500 mL
1 cup	diced peeled baking potatoes	250 mL
4 cups	chicken stock *or* vegetable stock *or* water	1 L
1 cup	fresh or frozen corn kernels	250 mL
1	red bell pepper, roasted (see Tip at left), peeled, seeded and diced	1
1	jalapeño pepper, seeded and chopped	1
	Black pepper	
1/4 cup	chopped fresh coriander or green onions or parsley	50 mL

1. In a large saucepan, heat oil over medium heat. Add onions and cook for 3 to 4 minutes or until softened but not browned. Add sweet potatoes and potatoes; cook for 2 to 3 minutes.

2. Add stock; bring to a boil. Reduce heat and simmer, uncovered, for 12 to 15 minutes or until potatoes are tender.

3. In a blender or food processor, purée potato mixture in batches; return to pan. Add corn, red pepper and jalapeño pepper. Cook for 3 to 4 minutes. Season to taste with salt and pepper. Serve soup garnished with coriander.

Complete the meal

Have with Best Hummus Dip (see recipe, page 49) and pita bread triangles or Pita Crisps (see recipe, page 48).

nutrient analysis

GRAIN PRODUCTS	VEGETABLES & FRUIT
	2

MILK PRODUCTS	MEAT & ALTERNATIVES

PER SERVING			
Calories	147	Carbohydrate	24 g
Protein	5.5 g	Dietary Fiber	2.8 g
Fat	3.7 g	Sodium	530 mg

Excellent source of vitamin A, vitamin C.
Good source of niacin.
Moderate source of dietary fiber.

SERVES 4

Tomato and Bean Soup

Marylin Cook
BRANTFORD, ON

P

MAKES 4 CUPS (1L)

This bright and tasty soup earned first-place honors at the Brant County Health Unit's "What's Cooking for Supper?" recipe contest. Ready in 15 minutes, it can be made in less time than it takes to order from a restaurant.

1	can (19 oz [540 mL]) stewed tomatoes	1
1	can (14 oz [398 mL]) baked beans in tomato sauce	1
1 cup	water	250 mL
1/2 cup	chopped onions	125 mL
1/2 tsp	dried basil	2 mL
1/2 tsp	dried parsley	2 mL
1 cup	shredded Cheddar cheese	250 mL

TIP

If you have fresh basil or parsley, use 1 tbsp (15 mL) or more of each instead of dried. You can also spice up the stewed tomatoes by adding 1 tsp (5 mL) Italian seasoning. If your kids don't like chunks of tomatoes or onions, purée them in a food processor or blender.

1. In a saucepan over medium heat, stir together tomatoes, beans, water, onions, basil and parsley; bring to a boil. Reduce heat to medium-low and simmer, uncovered and stirring occasionally, for 10 to 15 minutes.

2. Top each serving with 1/4 cup (50 mL) Cheddar cheese.

Complete the meal

Serve with whole wheat toast or bagels. Enjoy frozen yogurt for dessert.

Nutrition Facts

When you increase your fiber intake – as you will with this meal – be sure to drink more fluids.

food guide servings

GRAIN PRODUCTS	VEGETABLES & FRUIT
	1
1/2	1/2
MILK PRODUCTS	MEAT & ALTERNATIVES

nutrient analysis

PER SERVING			
Calories	259	Carbohydrate	33.5 g
Protein	13.8 g	Dietary Fiber	10.1 g
Fat	10.1 g	Sodium	971 mg

Excellent source of calcium, zinc. **Good** source of vitamin C, vitamin A, thiamin, niacin, folacin. **Very high** in dietary fiber.

SALADS AND VEGETABLES

Salads can be complete meals on their own or side dishes that add variety and extra nutrients to main meals. Look for "Complete the Meal" suggestions featured with each salad and vegetable side dish recipe.

what's in a serving?

One serving of vegetable or fruit is defined as 1 medium-sized vegetable or fruit (such as a banana, apple or potato) or 1/2 cup (125 mL) fresh, frozen or canned vegetables or fruit, 1 cup (250 mL) salad or 1/2 cup (125 mL) juice.

Remember your mother telling you to "eat your veggies"? Well, she was right! If you don't eat enough vegetables (or fruit) you could be missing out on nutrients and other substances that are important to your health. These foods also supply fiber (which is important in maintaining good health and a healthy weight) and, in most cases, they're naturally low in fat. Not surprisingly, *Canada's Food Guide to Healthy Eating* (see pages 176 to 177) recommends we have 5 to 10 servings of vegetables and fruit each day.

In this chapter you'll find salads suitable for main meals or for feeding a crowd. They're all easy to prepare – some simple enough for children to make. You'll also find some great vegetable side dishes that will add variety and nutrients to any meal.

Plant *power*

Vegetables and fruit are high in carbohydrates and fiber and a powerhouse of essential nutrients. They are particularly rich in vitamins A, C and folic acid. Some even provide small amounts of minerals, potassium (bananas, pears and oranges), iron (dried fruit and pumpkin) and calcium (kale, bok choy and mustard greens). But there's more:

Phytochemicals. These substances occur naturally in all plant foods including fruit, vegetables, legumes and grains. They are neither vitamins nor minerals and are calorie-free. They act as antioxidants and, as such, are thought to play a role in reducing the risk of chronic diseases such as heart disease and cancer.

Antioxidants. These compounds help to get rid of cell-damaging free radicals, which form in the body and get disease processes started. Antioxidants include vitamin C and beta-carotene (the plant form of vitamin A). Vitamin E is another antioxidant, which is found primarily in margarine and vegetable oils and, in smaller amounts, in leafy green vegetables, dried apricots, sweet potatoes, whole-grain cereals, wheat germ, nuts and seeds.

FIND THE PHYTOCHEMICALS

Phytochemical	Food Source
Carotenoids (such as beta carotene)	Orange and yellow fruits and vegetables, dark leafy greens
Carotenoids (such as lycopene)	Tomatoes
Flavonols (such as resveratrol)	Red grapes, red wine
Flavanones and carotenoids	Citrus fruits
Indoles, isothicyanates, carotenoids	Cruciferous vegetables (such as broccoli, cauliflower, brussels sprouts, kale and cabbage)
Isoflavanoids and phytosterols	Legumes, kidney and other beans, lentils, as well as soy products such as tofu

Source: "Beyond Vitamins: The New Nutrition Revolution," *UC Berkeley Wellness Letter,* April 1999.

Veggie variety

No single vegetable or fruit provides all the vitamins, minerals and phytochemicals that you need. So it's important to include a variety of vegetables and fruit in your daily meal plan.

Watch the *added* fat

While most vegetables and fruit are naturally low in fat, we often raise their fat content by cooking them in oil or by adding heavy dressings. Here are some suggestions for cutting that fat:

- Add flavor to vegetables and salads with herbs, lemon juice, flavored vinegars and low-fat salad dressing.

- Stir-fry vegetables with a minimum amount of oil.

- For vegetable dips and salads, cut the fat from creamy dressing by replacing half the salad dressing with lower-fat plain yogurt, yogurt cheese or creamed cottage cheese.

- Reduce the fat in vinaigrette salad dressing by replacing some of the oil with fruit juice or flavored vinegar (balsamic, rice wine or cider vinegar). Add a little bit of sugar to cut the tartness of the vinegar.

- Top baked potatoes with a mixture made from light sour cream and lower-fat plain yogurt or yogurt cheese. Add flavor with fresh herbs and chives.

- Make dips and salsas with fresh vegetables and fruit.

COLOR CODED

Go for color when choosing vegetables and fruit. The darker the color, the more nutrients and phytochemicals they contain.

Boost *those* servings

How can you eat the 5 to 10 servings of vegetables and fruit recommended in *Canada's Food Guide to Healthy Eating?* At first glance, it may seem a daunting task – particularly if, like many people, you eat most of your vegetables at dinner. The key is to add more vegetables and fruit to your diet throughout the day. Here are some suggestions.

- *Add fresh or canned fruit to your cereal, waffles, french toast or yogurt at breakfast.*

- *Take along fruit or raw veggies for quick snacks on the run.*

- *Have vegetable soup or salads, vegetable cocktail or tomato juice, or a piece of fruit with your lunch.*

- *Enjoy more servings of vegetables or fruit with your main meals.*

- *Instead of a rich dessert, have fruit as a fast finish to a meal.*

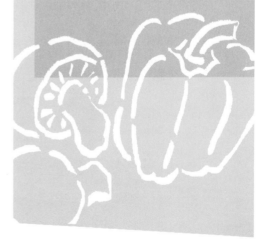

SERVES 6

Bev Callaghan, RD

Beet, Orange and Jicama Salad

MAKES 3 CUPS (750 mL)

Jicama is a crunchy, slightly sweet vegetable that tastes like a cross between a water chestnut and an apple. It adds a delicious crunch to this salad.

1	can (14 oz [398 mL]) sliced beets, drained	1
2	large navel oranges, peeled and cut into 1/4-inch (5 mm) slices	2
1/2 cup	thinly sliced sweet white onion	125 mL
1/2 cup	julienned jicama	125 mL

Dressing

2 tbsp	balsamic vinegar	25 mL
1 tbsp	orange juice	15 mL
1 tbsp	olive oil	15 mL
1/8 tsp	salt	0.5 mL
	Black pepper to taste	
1 tbsp	chopped fresh parsley (optional)	15 mL

Nutrition Facts

You can broaden your horizons – and your nutrient intake! – by trying a new vegetable each week. How about jicama, celeriac, rapini, kohlrabi or Swiss chard?

Complete the meal

This is a great winter salad to serve with soup and crusty bread or as an appetizer or side dish with a main meal.

1. In a medium bowl, combine beets, oranges, onions and jicama. Set aside.

2. In a small bowl, whisk together vinegar, orange juice, olive oil, salt and pepper. Add to beet mixture; toss gently. Chill. Sprinkle with parsley, if using, just before serving.

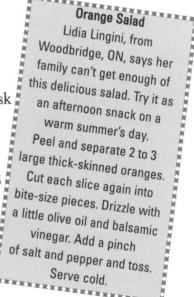

Orange Salad

Lidia Lingini, from Woodbridge, ON, says her family can't get enough of this delicious salad. Try it as an afternoon snack on a warm summer's day. Peel and separate 2 to 3 large thick-skinned oranges. Cut each slice again into bite-size pieces. Drizzle with a little olive oil and balsamic vinegar. Add a pinch of salt and pepper and toss. Serve cold.

food guide servings

GRAIN PRODUCTS	VEGETABLES & FRUIT
	1

MILK PRODUCTS	MEAT & ALTERNATIVES

nutrient analysis

PER SERVING			
Calories	71	Carbohydrate	12.4 g
Protein	1.2 g	Dietary Fiber	2.8 g
Fat	2.4 g	Sodium	174 mg

Excellent source of vitamin C. **Good** source of folacin. **Moderate** source of dietary fiber.

SERVES 4 | Chicken and Bean Salad

Lynn Homer, RD
Meals on Wheels
CALGARY, AB

P

MAKES 4 CUPS (1 L)

1	can (14 oz [398 mL]) kidney beans, rinsed and drained	1
1 cup	corn kernels, canned or frozen	250 mL
1 cup	cubed cooked chicken	250 mL
3/4 cup	diced red bell peppers	175 mL
2	green onions, chopped	2
1/4 cup	red wine vinegar	50 mL
2 tbsp	vegetable oil	25 mL
1/2 tsp	minced garlic	2 mL
1/4 tsp	salt	1 mL
1/4 tsp	black pepper	1 mL
1/4 to 1/2 tsp	hot pepper sauce (optional)	1 to 2 mL

1. In a medium bowl, combine beans, corn, chicken, peppers, onions, vinegar, oil, garlic, salt, pepper and, if using, hot pepper sauce. Toss gently until combined. Chill before serving.

Quick Marinated Bean Salad

This salad is great with burgers of any kind! It contains only 1.7 g fat and a whopping 10.2 g fiber per 1-cup (250 mL) serving. Cook 2 cups (500 mL) frozen cut green beans (or fresh, in season) until tender; drain and place in serving bowl. Add 1 can (19 oz [540 mL]) marinated bean salad (with liquid), 1/2 cup (125 mL) sliced red onions, 1 tbsp (15 mL) red wine vinegar, and a little sugar and pepper to taste. Toss.

Complete the meal

Pop some of this salad into half a pita bread or roll up in a flour tortilla. Have orange sherbet and digestive cookies for dessert.

food guide servings

GRAIN PRODUCTS	VEGETABLES & FRUIT
	1
	1
MILK PRODUCTS	MEAT & ALTERNATIVES

nutrient analysis

PER SERVING			
Calories	245	Carbohydrate	25.9 g
Protein	18.7 g	Dietary Fiber	7.2 g
Fat	8.3 g	Sodium	400 mg

Excellent source of vitamin C, niacin, vitamin B$_6$, folacin. **Very high** in dietary fiber.

SERVES 16

Coleslaw for a Crowd

Betty Walsh
OAKVILLE, ON

MAKES 12 CUPS (3 L)

This wonderful cabbage salad has been to more family gatherings than you can imagine, and is equally popular with children and adults. It's great for feeding a crowd and for pot-luck meals. If you don't have a crowd to feed, just cut the recipe in half.

8 cups	chopped green savoy cabbage	2 L
2 cups	chopped red apples (crisp or tart)	500 mL
1 1/2 cups	grated carrots	375 mL
1 1/2 cups	chopped celery	375 mL
1 cup	chopped green bell peppers	250 mL
1/2 cup	chopped green onions	125 mL
2/3 cup	light mayonnaise	150 mL
1 tsp	granulated sugar	5 mL
1/2 tsp	salt	2 mL

TIP

Regular cabbage can be used in place of the savoy cabbage. For best results, chop all ingredients by hand; using a food processor will make the salad too wet and mushy.

1. In a very large bowl, combine cabbage, apples, carrots, celery, green peppers and green onions.

2. In a small bowl or measuring cup, blend together mayonnaise, sugar and salt. Add to cabbage mixture; toss to blend well. Chill for 2 hours or overnight. (Don't worry if salad appears to need more dressing; after chilling, the mixture becomes creamier as the vegetables give off some juice.)

Make Ahead

You can buy the ingredients for this salad in advance and make it later in the week. Once made, the salad keeps well in the refrigerator for about 3 days.

Complete the meal

Serve with HOT 'N' SPICY TURKEY BURGERS (see recipe, page 131) or baked beans, cold cuts and rolls. Have ice cream for dessert.

food guide servings

GRAIN PRODUCTS	VEGETABLES & FRUIT
	1

MILK PRODUCTS	MEAT & ALTERNATIVES

nutrient analysis

PER SERVING			
Calories	58	Carbohydrate	7.4 g
Protein	1.0 g	Dietary Fiber	2.0 g
Fat	3.1 g	Sodium	161 mg

Excellent source of vitamin A. **Good** source of vitamin C, folacin. **Moderate** source of dietary fiber.

SERVES 10

Mary Sue Waisman, RD
CALGARY, AB

P

Colorful Bean and Corn Salad

MAKES (5 CUPS [1.25 L])

Let the kids toss some crunchy tortilla chips into the salad just before serving – then watch it disappear! Better yet, encourage older children to try making this salad on their own.

Food Fast

For a speedy dressing add 1/2 tsp (2 mL) cumin to 1/4 cup (50 mL) bottled oil-and-vinegar-type salad dressing.

Make Ahead

This salad is best made at least 4 to 6 hours or up to 1 day ahead to allow the flavors to blend. It keeps well in the refrigerator for up to 3 days.

Salad

1	can (19 oz [540 mL]) black beans, rinsed and drained	1
1	can (12 oz [341 mL]) corn kernels, drained	1
1 cup	chopped tomatoes	250 mL
1/2 cup	chopped green or red bell peppers	125 mL
1/2 cup	chopped red onions	125 mL
1/4 cup	chopped fresh parsley	50 mL

Dressing

2 tbsp	red wine vinegar *or* balsamic vinegar	25 mL
1 tbsp	olive oil	15 mL
1/2 tsp	ground cumin	2 mL
1/2 tsp	minced garlic	2 mL
1/2 tsp	hot pepper sauce (optional)	2 mL
1/4 tsp	salt	1 mL
	Black pepper	

1. In large bowl, combine beans, corn, tomatoes, peppers, onions and parsley. Set aside.

2. In a small bowl or measuring cup, whisk together vinegar, oil, cumin, garlic, hot pepper sauce (if using), salt and pepper to taste. Blend well. Pour over salad.

complete the meal

Serve topped with sliced black olives and crumbled feta cheese and whole grain bread or roll. Have sherbet and CRANBERRY OATMEAL COOKIES (see recipe, page 160) for dessert.

food guide servings

GRAIN PRODUCTS	VEGETABLES & FRUIT
	1/2
	1/2
MILK PRODUCTS	MEAT & ALTERNATIVES

nutrient analysis

PER SERVING			
Calories	94	Carbohydrate	16.9 g
Protein	4.4 g	Dietary Fiber	3.4 g
Fat	1.8 g	Sodium	230 mg

Excellent source of folacin. **Moderate** source of dietary fiber.

SERVES 6

Creamy Broccoli Salad

Adeline White
MANITOU, MB

MAKES ABOUT 5 CUPS (1.25 L)

This salad features a delicious dressing – just like the old-fashioned boiled dressings of long ago. Its flavor works particularly well with broccoli. The dressing is also terrific for coleslaw. Yum!

Nutrition Facts
Cruciferous vegetables such as broccoli, cauliflower, Brussels sprouts and rapini are rich in antioxidant vitamins and phytochemicals. Include them often in your diet. This salad is relatively high in fat, so don't make it an everyday meal.

Make Ahead
While best made on the day it is to be served, the salad and dressing can be prepared separately up to 1 day ahead. Toss salad with dressing just before serving.

Complete the meal
Serve with any grilled meat, fish or chicken and APRICOT BREAD PUDDING (see recipe, page 158) and a glass of milk.

Salad

4 1/2 cups	chopped broccoli (about 1 large head)	1.125 L
1 cup	quartered mushrooms	250 mL
4	slices cooked bacon, crumbled	4
1/2 cup	chopped red onions	125 mL
1/4 cup	toasted slivered almonds (see technique, page 124)	50 mL

Dressing

1	egg	1
2 tbsp	white wine vinegar	25 mL
2 tbsp	water	25 mL
2 tbsp	granulated sugar	25 mL
1/2 tsp	dry mustard	2 mL
1/2 tsp	cornstarch	2 mL
1/4 cup	light mayonnaise	50 mL

1. In a large pot of boiling water, blanch broccoli for no more than 2 minutes. Drain and refresh under cold water; drain again. Transfer to a large bowl. Add mushrooms, bacon, onions and almonds. Chill.

2. In a microwave-safe bowl, whisk together egg, vinegar, water, sugar, mustard and cornstarch. Microwave on High for 1 1/2 to 2 minutes, stirring at 30-second intervals. Set aside to cool. Blend in mayonnaise. Chill until ready to serve.

3. Just before serving, toss salad with dressing.

food guide servings

GRAIN PRODUCTS	VEGETABLES & FRUIT
	2
	1/4
MILK PRODUCTS	MEAT & ALTERNATIVES

nutrient analysis

PER SERVING			
Calories	142	Carbohydrate	11.7 g
Protein	5.8 g	Dietary Fiber	2.3 g
Fat	9.0 g	Sodium	162 mg

Excellent source of vitamin C. **Good** source of folacin. **Moderate** source of dietary fiber.

Erna Braun
WINNIPEG, MB

SERVES 6 Cucumber Raita Salad

MAKES 3 CUPS (750 ML)

This creamy salad is a perfect palate cooler to serve with any spicy meat or poultry dish.

To make 1 cup (250 mL) of yogurt cheese:
Use 2 cups (500 mL) of plain low-fat yogurt (balkan-style, not stirred, made without gelatin). Line a sieve with a double thickness of paper towel or cheesecloth. Pour yogurt into the sieve and place over a bowl. Cover well with plastic wrap and refrigerate for at least two hours. Discard liquid and keep in an airtight container in the refrigerator for up to a week.

If you want to drain overnight, use 3 cups (750 mL) yogurt to get 1 cup (250 mL) yogurt cheese. The longer you drain the yogurt the more tart it becomes. Yogurt cheese can be used in a variety of other dips and dressings.

3 cups	thinly sliced English cucumber, unpeeled (about 1 large)	750 mL
1/2 tsp	salt	2 mL
1/2 cup	yogurt cheese (for technique, see left)	125 mL
1/2 tsp	lemon juice	2 mL
1/4 tsp	minced garlic	1 mL
1/4 tsp	ground ginger	1 mL

1. Place cucumber slices in a large colander; sprinkle with salt. Let stand for 10 to 15 minutes over a large bowl (or in the sink) to drain. Rinse well under cold water. Pat dry and transfer to a bowl. Set aside.

2. In a separate bowl, blend together yogurt cheese, lemon juice, garlic and ginger. Add mixture to cucumbers; toss gently. Chill before serving.

Complete the meal
Serve with CURRIED RED PEPPER CHICKEN (see recipe, page 130) and rice.

food guide servings

GRAIN PRODUCTS	VEGETABLES & FRUIT
	1/2
1/4	
MILK PRODUCTS	MEAT & ALTERNATIVES

nutrient analysis

PER 1/2 CUP 125 ML SERVING			
Calories	27	Carbohydrate	3.4 g
Protein	2.3 g	Dietary Fiber	0.4 g
Fat	0.6 g	Sodium	19 mg

SERVES 4

Jane Bellman, RD
HAMILTON, ON

Fast and Easy Greek Salad

MAKES 6 CUPS (1.5 L)

Here's a simple salad that's sure to please. It's especially great when fresh local tomatoes are in season.

Nutrition Facts
This salad is higher in fat, so it's best served with lower-fat dishes. If you don't have time to make the dressing, use a bottled oil-and-vinegar type dressing. Choose a dressing that contains less than 3 g fat per 1 tbsp (15 mL) to help cut the fat.

2 cups	diced tomatoes	500 mL
2 cups	diced cucumbers	500 mL
1 cup	cubed feta cheese (about 8 oz [250 g])	250 mL
1/2 cup	thinly sliced onions	125 mL
1/4 cup	sliced black olives (optional)	50 mL
2 tbsp	white wine vinegar	25 mL
2 tbsp	olive oil	25 mL
1/2 tsp	minced garlic	2 mL
1/2 tsp	dried basil	2 mL
1/2 tsp	dried oregano	2 mL
	Black pepper	

1. In a large bowl, combine tomatoes, cucumbers, cheese, onions and, if using, olives. Set aside.

2. In a small bowl or measuring cup, whisk together vinegar, oil, garlic, basil, oregano and pepper. Add to tomato mixture; toss gently to combine. Chill before serving.

Complete the meal

Serve with BARBECUED BUTTERFLIED LEG OF LAMB (see recipe, page 116) and pita bread.

food guide servings

GRAIN PRODUCTS	VEGETABLES & FRUIT
	1 1/2
1/2	
MILK PRODUCTS	MEAT & ALTERNATIVES

nutrient analysis

PER SERVING			
Calories	177	Carbohydrate	9.3 g
Protein	5.8 g	Dietary Fiber	1.8 g
Fat	13.8 g	Sodium	357 mg

Excellent source of vitamin B$_{12}$. **Good** source of vitamin C, riboflavin, folacin, calcium.

SERVES 6

Fusilli and Fruit Salad

Josie Haresign
WINNIPEG, MB

P

MAKES 6 CUPS (1.5 L)

Here's an unusual salad that even the fussiest of kids will enjoy.

If you like things spicy, add 1 tsp (5 mL) curry powder to the yogurt cheese.

TIP

Try using a variety of different fruits. You will need about 4 cups (1 L) in total.

Make Ahead

Salad can be made a day ahead. Prepare salad and dressing separately and combine just before serving.

1 1/2 cups	fusilli (spiral pasta)	375 mL
1	can (14 oz [398 mL]) pineapple tidbits, drained	1
1	can (10 oz [284 mL]) whole mandarin orange segments, drained	1
1 cup	halved red or green grapes	250 mL
1/2 cup	diced unpeeled red apples	125 mL
1/2 cup	yogurt cheese (for technique, see page 85) *or* lower-fat thick yogurt	125 mL
2 tbsp	frozen orange juice concentrate, thawed	25 mL
1	small banana, sliced	1

1. In a pot of boiling water, cook pasta until tender but firm; drain. Rinse under cold water; drain. Transfer to a large bowl. Add pineapple, oranges, grapes and apples.

2. In a separate bowl, stir together yogurt cheese and orange juice concentrate. Pour over pasta mixture; toss gently. Chill. Stir in sliced banana just before serving.

Complete the meal

This salad is great served with cold cooked chicken legs.

GRAIN PRODUCTS	VEGETABLES & FRUIT
1/2	1 1/2
1/4	
MILK PRODUCTS	MEAT & ALTERNATIVES

nutrient analysis

PER SERVING			
Calories	198	Carbohydrate	43.2 g
Protein	5.5 g	Dietary Fiber	2.5 g
Fat	1.3 g	Sodium	21 mg

Excellent source of folacin. **Good** source of vitamin C, thiamin, riboflavin. **Moderate** source of dietary fiber.

SERVES 8

Carol Ermanovics
NEPEAN, ON

German Potato Salad Picnic-Style

MAKES 8 CUPS (2 L)

This creamy potato salad contains only 3.8 g fat per 1-cup (250 mL) serving. Take it along on your next picnic – just be sure to keep it cold in an insulated cooler with lots of ice packs, and keep your cooler in the shade!

Foods that sit out for more than 2 hours in the heat – or even at room temperature – should be discarded. In these conditions, bacteria multiply quickly, particularly on high-risk foods such as meats, dairy products, salads and sandwiches.

TIP

While potatoes are cooking, add a large sprig of rosemary, thyme or tarragon to the water to increase their flavor.

Make Ahead
You can prepare the salad through Step 2 up to 1 day ahead. Chill.

3 lbs	small red new potatoes, halved or quartered	1.5 kg
1/4 cup	white wine vinegar	50 mL
1 tbsp	granulated sugar	15 mL
1/2 tsp	salt	2 mL
1/4 tsp	celery seed	1 mL
1/4 tsp	black pepper	1 mL
6	green onions, chopped	6
2 tbsp	chopped fresh dill (or 1 tsp [5 mL] dried)	25 mL
3/4 cup	light (5%) sour cream	175 mL
1 tsp	Dijon mustard	5 mL
4	hard-boiled eggs	4

1. In a large saucepan, gently boil potatoes for 12 to 15 minutes or until tender but still firm; drain. Transfer to a large bowl.

2. In a microwave-safe measuring cup, combine vinegar, sugar, salt, celery seed and pepper. Microwave on High for 30 seconds or until very hot; pour over warm potatoes. Stir gently until vinegar is absorbed. Add onions and dill to potatoes.

3. In the same measuring cup, stir together sour cream and mustard. Fold gently into potato mixture. Chill.

4. Just before serving, cut hard-boiled eggs into quarters. Place 2 quarters with each serving of salad.

complete the meal
Take on a picnic with bean salad, rolls, cold cuts, cheese slices and fruit.

food guide servings

GRAIN PRODUCTS	VEGETABLES & FRUIT
	2
	1/2
MILK PRODUCTS	MEAT & ALTERNATIVES

nutrient analysis

PER SERVING			
Calories	196	Carbohydrate	33.7 g
Protein	7.6 g	Dietary Fiber	2.6 g
Fat	3.8 g	Sodium	212 mg

Excellent source of vitamin B$_6$. **Good** source of vitamin C, niacin. **Moderate** source of dietary fiber.

SERVES 4

Mandarin Orange Salad with Almonds

Evelyn Witt
ASSINIBOIA, SK

P

Evelyn serves this salad as part of an Easter brunch – to rave reviews. But you can serve it at any time, since all of the ingredients are readily available throughout the year.

Food Fast
Don't have time to wash salad greens? Plan ahead: instead of washing only the greens you need, wash a whole head of lettuce or a bag of spinach. Toss in a salad spinner to remove extra moisture. Store lettuce in the salad spinner or wrapped in paper towels in a plastic bag until needed.

Allergy Alert
Check to see if anyone has nut allergies before using almonds in this recipe.

To make candied almonds:
In a small nonstick skillet, melt 1 tbsp (15 mL) sugar over low heat. Add 1/4 cup (50 mL) slivered almonds and cook, stirring constantly, for 5 to 6 minutes or until almonds are well coated with syrup and lightly browned. Cool; break apart into small pieces.

8 cups	torn romaine lettuce leaves	2 L
1/2 cup	sliced celery	125 mL
2	green onions, chopped	2
1	can (10 oz [284 mL]) mandarin orange segments, drained	1

Dressing

2 tbsp	vinegar	25 mL
4 tsp	olive oil	20 mL
1 tbsp	chopped fresh parsley (or 1 tsp [5 mL] dried)	15 mL
2 tsp	granulated sugar	10 mL
1/4 tsp	hot pepper sauce	1 mL
1/4 tsp	salt	1 mL
	Black pepper	
	Candied almonds (see instructions, lower left)	

1. In a large bowl, combine lettuce, celery, onions and mandarin oranges. Set aside.

2. Dressing: In a small bowl, whisk together vinegar, oil, parsley, sugar, hot pepper sauce and salt. Season to taste with pepper. Pour over salad; toss to coat. Serve sprinkled with candied almonds.

complete the meal
Try this salad with TUNA AND RICE CASSEROLE (see recipe, page 144).

GRAIN PRODUCTS	VEGETABLES & FRUIT
	2 1/2
	1/4
MILK PRODUCTS	MEAT & ALTERNATIVES

nutrient analysis

PER SERVING			
Calories	166	Carbohydrate	20.1 g
Protein	4.0 g	Dietary Fiber	3.2 g
Fat	9.0 g	Sodium	171 mg

Excellent source of vitamin A, vitamin C, folacin. **Moderate** source of dietary fiber.

SERVES 8

Marguerite McDuff
ST. LOUIS DE BLANDFORD, PQ

Penne Salad with Asparagus and Tuna

MAKES 10 CUPS (2.5 L)

This makes a delicious main-dish salad. The ginger adds a unique taste.

Nutrition Facts

For best flavor and nutrients, buy fresh vegetables locally and in season. When asparagus is out of season, use green beans or broccoli instead.

Make Ahead

Prepare salad and dressing separately. Chill for up to 1 day. Toss salad with dressing just before serving.

Complete the meal

Serve this salad with some milk or cheese and you'll have a meal that includes all four food groups.

3 cups	penne (about 10 oz [300 g])	750 mL
3 cups	fresh asparagus, trimmed and cut into bite-size pieces, (about 1 lb [500 g])	750 mL
2	cans (each 5.7 oz [170 g]) water-packed tuna, drained	2
1 cup	diced red bell peppers	250 mL
2 tbsp	chopped chives or green onions	25 mL
2 tbsp	capers, drained (optional)	25 mL

Dressing

2 tbsp	balsamic vinegar *or* red wine vinegar	25 mL
2 tbsp	olive oil	25 mL
2 tsp	Dijon mustard	10 mL
1 tsp	brown sugar	5 mL
1/2 tsp	minced garlic	2 mL
1/2 tsp	minced ginger root	2 mL
	Salt	
	Black pepper	

1. In a large pot of boiling water, cook penne according to package directions or until tender but firm, adding asparagus during last 2 minutes of cooking time; drain. Rinse under cold water; drain. Transfer to a large bowl. Add tuna, peppers, chives and, if using, capers. Set aside.

2. Dressing: In a small bowl or measuring cup, whisk together vinegar, oil, mustard, sugar, garlic and ginger. Season to taste with salt and pepper. Pour over salad; toss gently to combine. Serve immediately.

food guide servings

GRAIN PRODUCTS	VEGETABLES & FRUIT
1 1/2	1
	1/2
MILK PRODUCTS	MEAT & ALTERNATIVES

nutrient analysis

PER SERVING			
Calories	223	Carbohydrate	30.9 g
Protein	14.4 g	Dietary Fiber	2.5 g
Fat	4.6 g	Sodium	137 mg

Excellent source of niacin, folacin, vitamin B$_{12}$. **Good** source of iron, vitamin C, thiamin, riboflavin. **Moderate** source of fiber.

Roasted Red Pepper Salad

Nikola Ajdacic
TORONTO, ON

P

For a beautiful presentation, arrange pepper slices on a round platter with their edges overlapping in a circular pattern. Garnish with a large sprig of fresh basil in the center. For a little added spice, sprinkle with a dash of cayenne pepper and crushed garlic.

6	roasted red bell peppers, each cut into 6 strips	6
1 tbsp	balsamic vinegar *or* red wine vinegar	15 mL
2 tsp	olive oil	10 mL
2 tbsp	chopped fresh basil (or 1 tsp [5 mL] dried), optional	25 mL
	Freshly ground black pepper	

1. Arrange peppers in the bottom of a shallow serving dish. Set aside.

2. In a small bowl or measuring cup, whisk together vinegar and olive oil; drizzle over peppers. Sprinkle with basil, if using. Season to taste with pepper. Chill for at least 1 hour before serving.

TIP

Keep roasted red peppers in your freezer and you can make this salad anytime. For instructions on roasting peppers, see QUICK ROASTED RED PEPPER DIP (page 51).

Throughout much of the year, red peppers tend to be expensive. Before buying, weigh peppers of equal size in your hand and choose the lighter ones. Heavier peppers have more seeds, which you end up paying for but not eating.

Nutrition Facts
Red peppers are rich in phytochemicals and antioxidants such as beta-carotene and vitamin C.

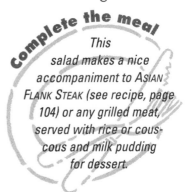

Complete the meal

This salad makes a nice accompaniment to ASIAN FLANK STEAK (see recipe, page 104) or any grilled meat, served with rice or couscous and milk pudding for dessert.

nutrient analysis

GRAIN PRODUCTS	VEGETABLES & FRUIT
	2
MILK PRODUCTS	MEAT & ALTERNATIVES

PER SERVING			
Calories	48	Carbohydrate	8.3 g
Protein	1.1 g	Dietary Fiber	1.7 g
Fat	1.7 g	Sodium	2 mg

Excellent source of vitamin A, vitamin C. **Good** source of vitamin B$_6$.

SERVES 4

Colette Villeneuve
VAL BELAIR, PQ

This main-meal salad makes a great summer supper when fresh vegetables and herbs are in season.

TIP

Try replacing the salmon with canned tuna packed in water.

Nutrition Facts

For added nutrients and fiber, leave the skins on the potatoes. Don't use potatoes that have a greenish tinge; this is caused by overexposure to light, which increases levels of a bitter compound called solanin. Eating green potatoes can cause a stomach upset.

Salmon, Potato and Green Bean Salad

MAKES 5 CUPS (1.25 L)

1 lb	small new white potatoes, halved or quartered	500 g
1 cup	green beans, cut into 2-inch (5 cm) pieces	250 mL
1	green onion, chopped	1
1 cup	halved cherry tomatoes or diced tomatoes	250 mL
2 tbsp	chopped fresh basil (or 1 tsp [5 mL] dried)	25 mL
1/3 cup	bottled oil-and-vinegar-type dressing	75 mL
2	cans (each 7 1/2 oz [213 g]) salmon, drained, bones and skin removed	2
	Salt	
	Black pepper	

1. In a medium saucepan, gently boil potatoes for 10 to 15 minutes or until tender but firm, adding beans during last 4 minutes of cooking time. Drain and transfer vegetables to a large bowl.

2. Add green onion, tomatoes and basil. Add dressing; toss gently to combine. Gently stir in salmon. Season to taste with salt and pepper. Chill before serving.

Complete the me

Add a light finish to the meal with store-boug angel food cake, topp with a mixture of van. yogurt and fruit.

food guide servings

GRAIN PRODUCTS	VEGETABLES & FRUIT
	2
	1
MILK PRODUCTS	MEAT & ALTERNATIVES

nutrient analysis

PER SERVING			
Calories	295	Carbohydrate	25.3 g
Protein	18.9 g	Dietary Fiber	2.5 g
Fat	13.5 g	Sodium	666 mg

Excellent source of niacin, vitamin B$_6$, vitamin B$_{12}$. **Good** source of vitamin C, folacin, iron. **Moderate** source of dietary fiber.

Lorraine Fullum-Bouchard, RD
OTTAWA, ON

SERVES 6

Triple-Bean Salad with Rice and Artichokes

MAKES 6 CUPS (1.5 L)

This salad is a snap to make because the dressing comes with the marinated beans! It also makes a great picnic lunch. As Lorraine says, "this is very tasty wrapped in a flour tortilla or in pita bread."

TIP

Try experimenting with different grains in salads. Good choices include brown rice, couscous, bulgur and quinoa.

If using quinoa, rinse well before cooking to remove the bitter outer coating.

2 cups	cooked rice or quinoa	500 mL
1	can (19 oz [540 mL]) marinated bean salad, with liquid	1
1	can (14 oz [398 mL]) artichoke hearts, drained and diced	1
1 cup	diced seeded plum tomatoes	250 mL
4	green onions, chopped	4
1/4 cup	chopped fresh parsley (optional)	50 mL
1 tbsp	white wine vinegar	15 mL
1 tsp	minced garlic	5 mL
1 tsp	dried oregano	5 mL
1/2 tsp	black pepper	2 mL

1. In a large bowl, combine rice, bean salad, artichokes, tomatoes, onions and, if using, parsley. Add vinegar, garlic, oregano and pepper; toss to combine. Chill before serving.

Complete the meal
Serve this salad topped with some cubed feta cheese or have it with a glass of milk.

food guide servings

GRAIN PRODUCTS	VEGETABLES & FRUIT
1/2	1
	1/2
MILK PRODUCTS	MEAT & ALTERNATIVES

nutrient analysis

PER SERVING			
Calories	216	Carbohydrate	36.6 g
Protein	7.9 g	Dietary Fiber	6.7 g
Fat	5.1 g	Sodium	201 mg

Excellent source of folacin. **Very high** in dietary fiber.

SERVES 6

Gaitree Peters
GUELPH, ON

Vietnamese Chicken and Rice Noodle Salad

MAKES ABOUT 8 CUPS (2 L)

Vietnamese fish sauce (nuoc mam) is an integral part of Vietnamese cooking. It is a clear, pungent liquid made by fermenting fish with salt. It takes a little getting used to! Fish sauce is high in sodium, so use it sparingly. Look in the specialty foods section of some supermarkets.

3 1/2 oz	wide rice noodles (Half a 7-oz [210 g] package)	99 g
12 oz	shredded cooked chicken	375 g
2 cups	diced cucumbers	500 mL
2 cups	shredded carrots	500 mL
1 cup	julienned green bell peppers	250 mL
1/4 cup	finely chopped cilantro	50 mL

Dressing

1/3 cup	fish sauce *or* sodium-reduced soya sauce	75 mL
1/4 cup	rice wine vinegar	50 mL
2 tbsp	lime juice	25 mL
1 to 2 tbsp	curry paste	15 to 25 mL
2 tsp	granulated sugar	10 mL
1 tsp	minced garlic	5 mL
1 tsp	sesame oil	5 mL
1/2 cup	chopped peanuts (optional)	125 mL

Food Fast

To ensure a ready supply of cooked chicken for recipes like this one, cook whole chickens when you have time on the weekend. Cut up and freeze in 1-cup (250 mL) portions to use as needed.

Complete the meal

Have this salad with a serving of fruit-flavored yogurt to increase your intake of calcium.

1. In a large pot of boiling water, cook noodles for 5 to 8 minutes or until barely tender; drain. Rinse under cold water; drain. Transfer to a large bowl. Add chicken, cucumbers, carrots, peppers and cilantro.

2. Dressing: In a small bowl, blend together soya sauce, vinegar, lime juice, curry paste, sugar, garlic and sesame oil. Add dressing to noodle mixture; toss to combine. Sprinkle with peanuts, if using.

food guide servings

GRAIN PRODUCTS	VEGETABLES & FRUIT
1/2	1
	1
MILK PRODUCTS	MEAT & ALTERNATIVES

nutrient analysis

PER SERVING			
Calories	214	Carbohydrate	23.1 g
Protein	19.4 g	Dietary Fiber	1.8 g
Fat	4.8 g	Sodium	594 mg

Excellent source of vitamin A, niacin, vitamin B$_6$. **Good** source of vitamin C, zinc.

SERVES 6 | Cauliflower Casserole

Dairy Farmers of Canada

This casserole is simple to prepare, yet elegant enough for entertaining. You can replace the cauliflower with broccoli or use a combination of broccoli and cauliflower.

6 cups	cauliflower florets	1.5 L
1 tbsp	butter	15 mL
2 tbsp	flour	25 mL
1/2 tsp	dry mustard	2 mL
1 1/4 cups	milk	300 mL
1 cup	grated Swiss or Cheddar cheese	250 mL
1/4 tsp	salt	1 mL
1/4 tsp	black pepper	1 mL
1/2 cup	corn flake-type cereal crumbs	125 mL
2 tsp	butter, melted	10 mL

Food Fast

If you don't have the 20 to 25 minutes needed to make this casserole, you can always cook up a bowl of steamed fresh cauliflower or broccoli (or a combination of both) in the microwave. They'll cook up in about 3 to 4 minutes on High per 8 oz (250 g). Add about 1 tbsp (15 mL) water and cover the dish with a plate so that the vegetables will steam themselves. Let stand for 1 to 2 minutes before serving.

Nutrition Facts

To keep your fat intake in balance, serve higher-fat vegetable dishes such as this one with lower-fat main meals.

Make Ahead

Casserole can be made up to one day ahead and refrigerated. Remove from fridge 30 minutes before baking and increase baking time by about 5 minutes.

1. In a large saucepan, cook cauliflower in boiling water for 3 to 4 minutes or until just barely tender-crisp; drain and place in prepared baking dish.

2. In another saucepan, melt butter over medium heat; stir in flour and mustard. Whisk in milk and cook, stirring constantly, until mixture boils and thickens. Remove from heat; stir in cheese. Add salt and pepper. Pour mixture evenly over cauliflower.

3. In a small bowl, combine crumbs and butter; sprinkle over top of cauliflower mixture. Bake in pre-heated oven for 10 to 15 minutes or until heated through.

complete the meal

Serve as a side dish with any grilled or broiled meat such as ASIAN FLANK STEAK (see recipe, page 104), or BROILED HAM STEAK WITH PINEAPPLE-MANGO SALSA (see recipe, page 115).

nutrient analysis

GRAIN PRODUCTS	VEGETABLES & FRUIT
1/2	2
1/4	
MILK PRODUCTS	MEAT & ALTERNATIVES

PER SERVING			
Calories	193	Carbohydrate	17.8 g
Protein	9.9 g	Dietary Fiber	2.1 g
Fat	9.6 g	Sodium	301 mg

Excellent source of vitamin C, folacin, calcium. **Good** source of thiamin, niacin, vitamin B_6, vitamin B_{12}. **Moderate** source of dietary fiber.

SERVES 8

Easy Scalloped Potatoes

Eileen Gibson
TORONTO, ON

P

These are the easiest, most delicious scalloped potatoes you will ever make!

TIP

To speed up preparation time, buy pre-grated cheese or have a handy youngster do it for you.

Food Fast

Looking for baked potatoes in a hurry? Use your microwave! A medium potato (6 to 8 oz [175 to 250 g]) takes only 3 to 4 minutes to cook on High. Pierce with a fork before cooking. Let stand for 2 minutes to soften before serving. Alternatively, you can start baked potatoes in the microwave and crisp them up in a toaster oven or on the barbecue.

PREHEAT OVEN TO 325° F (160° C)
13- BY 9-INCH (3 L) BAKING DISH, GREASED

1	can (10 oz [284 mL]) condensed cream of celery soup	1
1 1/4 cups	milk (1 full soup can)	300 mL
1/2 cup	sliced onions	125 mL
3 cups	potatoes, cut into slices 1/4 inch (5 mm) thick	750 mL
1/2 cup	grated Cheddar cheese	125 mL
	Black pepper	
	Paprika	

1. In a large bowl, stir together soup, milk, onions and potatoes. Pour into prepared baking dish; sprinkle with cheese. Season to taste with pepper and paprika. Bake for 65 to 75 minutes or until potatoes are tender.

Complete the meal

Serve with BROILED HAM STEAK WITH PINEAPPLE-MANGO SALSA (see recipe, page 115) and PEAR GINGERBREAD UPSIDE-DOWN CAKE (see recipe, page 170).

food guide servings

GRAIN PRODUCTS	VEGETABLES & FRUIT
	1
1/4	
MILK PRODUCTS	MEAT & ALTERNATIVES

nutrient analysis

PER SERVING			
Calories	149	Carbohydrate	21.9 g
Protein	5.0 g	Dietary Fiber	1.5 g
Fat	4.8 g	Sodium	353 mg

VEGGIE, BEEF AND PASTA BAKE (PAGE 114) ➤
OVERLEAF: POLYNESIAN PORK KEBABS (PAGE 118)

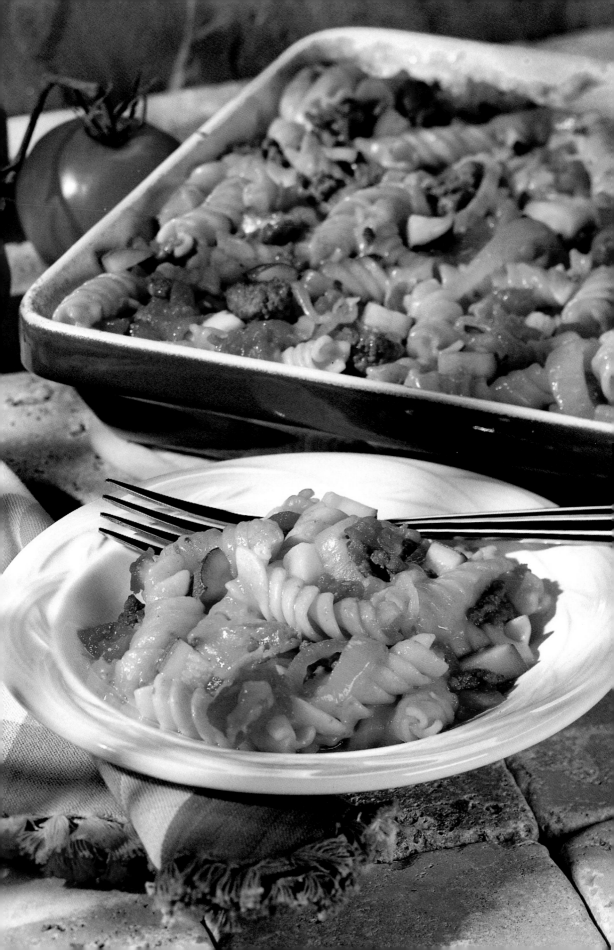

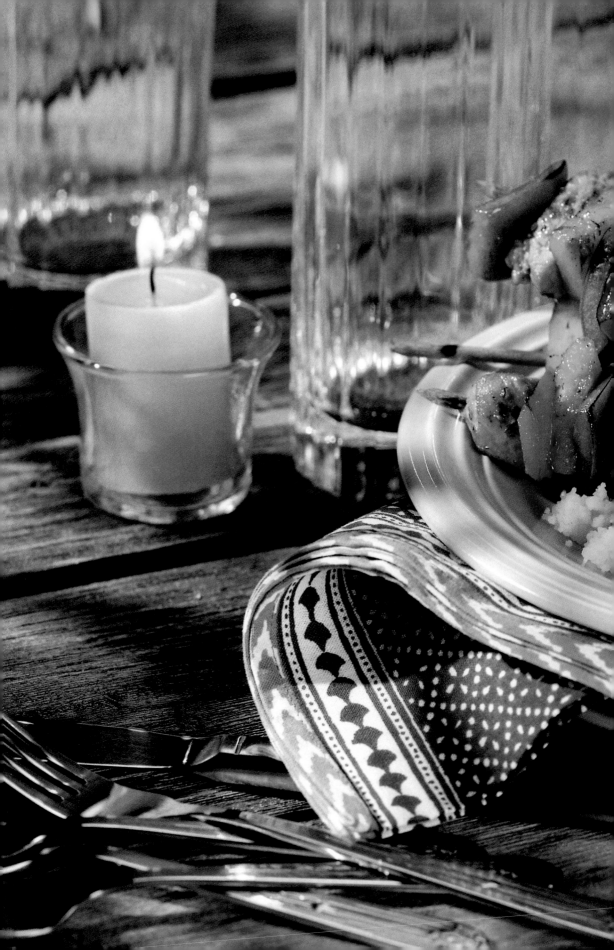

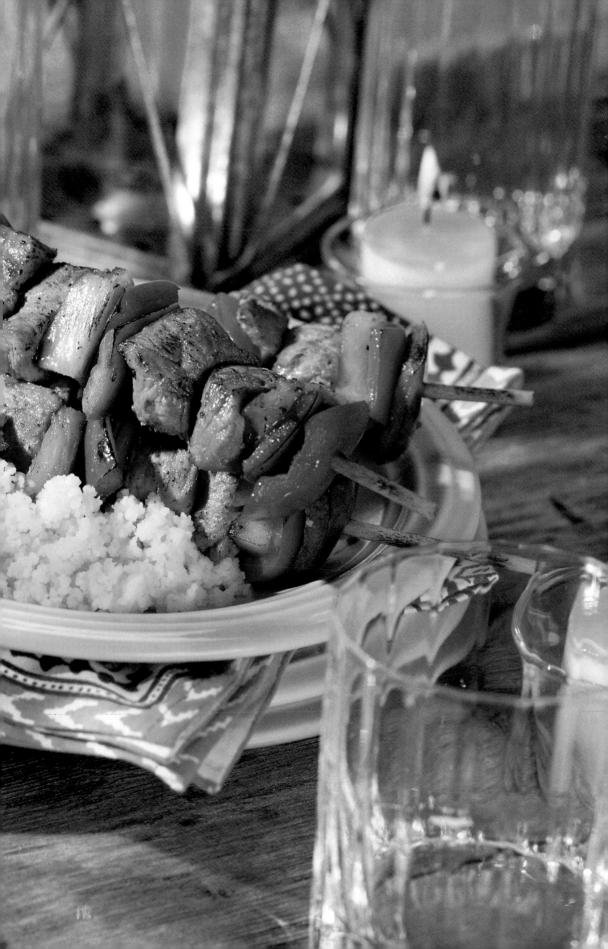

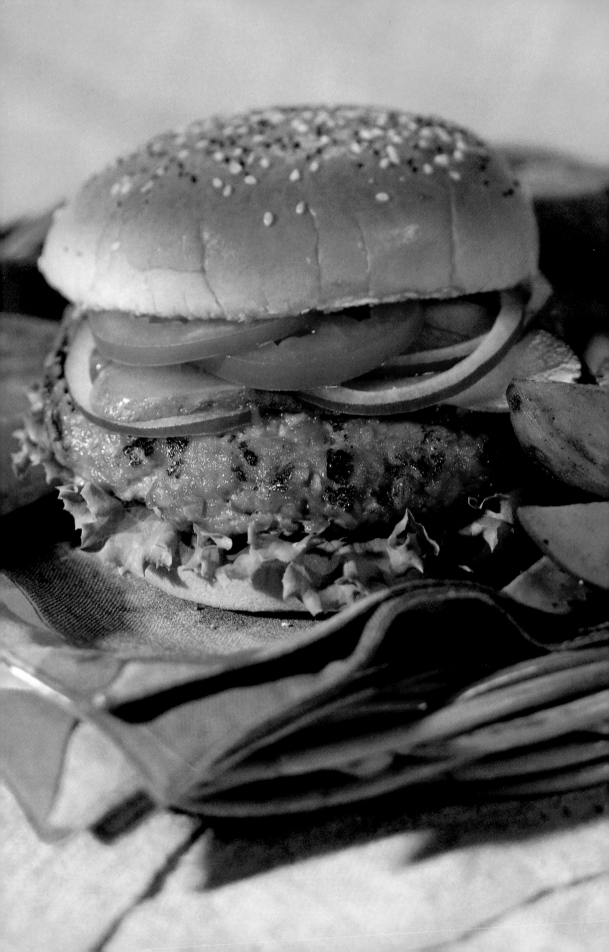

Honey-Glazed Carrots

SERVES 4

Lynn Roblin, RD

P

Get children involved in helping with grating carrots and other food preparation jobs. When children have had a hand in preparing a food they are more likely to eat it.

Some children find cooked carrots bitter – if that's the case with your kids, hold some back and serve them raw.

1 lb	carrots, cut into 1-inch (2.5 cm) pieces	500 g
1 tbsp	liquid honey *or* brown sugar	15 mL
1 tbsp	orange juice	15 mL
2 tsp	butter *or* margarine	10 mL
1/2 tsp	ground ginger	2 mL
1/2 tsp	grated orange zest (optional)	2 mL

1. In a medium saucepan over high heat, boil carrots until tender-crisp; drain. Add honey, orange juice, butter, ginger and, if using, zest. Quickly stir for 2 to 3 minutes or until glaze forms.

food guide servings

GRAIN PRODUCTS	VEGETABLES & FRUIT
	1 1/2
MILK PRODUCTS	MEAT & ALTERNATIVES

nutrient analysis

PER SERVING			
Calories	77	Carbohydrate	14.6 g
Protein	1.1 g	Dietary Fiber	2.5 g
Fat	2.1 g	Sodium	81 mg

Excellent source of vitamin A. **Moderate** source of dietary fiber.

Sweet Potato "Fries"

SERVES 4

Bev Callaghan, RD

PREHEAT OVEN TO 375° F (190° C)
NONSTICK BAKING SHEET

Here's a delicious alternative to French fries – with more nutrients and less fat.

Food Fast
For a super-quick sweet potato, cook it in the microwave. Just scrub a medium (8 oz [250 g]) potato, pierce it with a fork and microwave on High for 2 to 3 minutes. Let stand for 2 minutes before serving.

1 lb	sweet potatoes, each cut lengthwise into 6 wedges	500 g
2 tsp	vegetable oil	10 mL
1/4 tsp	paprika	1 mL
1/8 tsp	garlic powder	0.5 mL
	Black pepper	

1. Place potatoes in a bowl. Add oil, paprika and garlic powder. Season to taste with pepper. Toss to coat. Transfer to baking sheet. Bake for 25 minutes or until tender and golden, turning once.

food guide servings

GRAIN PRODUCTS	VEGETABLES & FRUIT
	1
MILK PRODUCTS	MEAT & ALTERNATIVES

nutrient analysis

PER SERVING			
Calories	105	Carbohydrate	20.0 g
Protein	1.4 g	Dietary Fiber	2.5 g
Fat	2.4 g	Sodium	8 mg

Excellent source of vitamin A. **Good** source of vitamin C. **Moderate** source of dietary fiber.

◄ HOT 'N' SPICY TURKEY BURGERS (PAGE 131)

Roasted Carrots and Parsnips

SERVES 8

Bev Callaghan, RD

P

The maple syrup in this recipe makes sweet-tasting vegetables that even children will enjoy.

Food Fast

For a quick vegetable fix, cut a fresh tomato in half; sprinkle with dry bread crumbs, dried herbs and Parmesan cheese. Bake at 350° F (180° C) for 20 minutes as you prepare the rest of dinner.

PREHEAT OVEN TO 400° F (200° C)
13- BY 9-INCH (3 L) BAKING PAN, GREASED

1 lb	parsnips, peeled and cut into 1-inch (2.5 cm) pieces	500 g
1 lb	carrots, peeled and cut into 1-inch (2.5 cm) pieces	500 g
1 cup	onions, cut into wedges	250 mL
2 tbsp	vegetable oil	25 mL
1 tsp	dried thyme	5 mL
2 tbsp	maple syrup	25 mL
1 tbsp	Dijon mustard	15 mL

1. Place parsnips, carrots, onions, oil and thyme in prepared baking dish; toss until vegetables are well coated with oil. Roast in oven for 30 minutes.

2. Meanwhile, in a small bowl, combine maple syrup and mustard. Pour over vegetables; toss to coat. Roast for another 20 to 25 minutes or until vegetables are tender and golden, stirring once.

Complete the meal

This dish is delicious with PARMESAN-HERB BAKED FISH FILLETS (see recipe, page 138), a crusty roll and ORANGE CRÈME CARAMEL (see recipe, page 168).

food guide servings

GRAIN PRODUCTS	VEGETABLES & FRUIT
	1 1/2
MILK PRODUCTS	MEAT & ALTERNATIVES

nutrient analysis

PER SERVING			
Calories	113	Carbohydrate	19.7 g
Protein	1.5 g	Dietary Fiber	3.2 g
Fat	3.8 g	Sodium	62 mg

Excellent source of vitamin A. **Good** source of folacin. **Moderate** source of dietary fiber.

Sautéed Spinach with Pine Nuts

Bev Callaghan, RD

This is a great way to jazz up plain spinach. You can easily substitute Swiss chard, kale, rapini, or mustard greens for the spinach.

TIP
Stir-frying vegetables is a great way to preserve nutrients. When boiled, vegetables can lose of up to 45% of vitamin C compared to losing only 5% when stir-fried.

Nutrition Facts
Women who are pregnant or planning a pregnancy need more iron and folacin in their diet. This dish can help increase intakes of both.

Allergy Alert
This dish contains nuts, so check for nut allergies before serving to guests.

2 tsp	olive oil	10 mL
1/4 cup	pine nuts	50 mL
1	package (10 oz [300 g]) fresh spinach, trimmed of tough stalks	1
1 tsp	minced garlic	5 mL
1 tsp	lemon juice	5 mL
1/8 tsp	nutmeg	0.5 mL
	Black pepper	

1. In a large nonstick skillet, heat 1 tsp (5 mL) of the oil over medium heat. Add pine nuts and cook, stirring constantly, for 2 to 3 minutes or until golden. Remove pine nuts from pan and set aside.

2. Add remaining oil to pan. Add spinach in several bunches (it will cook down quickly), stirring constantly. Add garlic and cook for 1 to 2 minutes. Stir in lemon juice and nutmeg. Season to taste with pepper. Add reserved pine nuts. Cook until heated through.

Complete the meal
Serve with any grilled or baked meat, fish or poultry, whole-grain bread and a milk-based dessert.

GRAIN PRODUCTS	VEGETABLES & FRUIT
	1
	1/4
MILK PRODUCTS	MEAT & ALTERNATIVES

nutrient analysis

PER SERVING			
Calories	90	Carbohydrate	4.4 g
Protein	4.5 g	Dietary Fiber	3.3 g
Fat	7.6 g	Sodium	48 mg

Excellent source of vitamin A, folacin. **Good** source of iron. **Moderate** source of dietary fiber.

Main Meals

MAIN MEALS

Pick your *protein*

The recipes in this chapter help satisfy some of your daily protein requirements. In order to benefit from the various nutrients that different protein foods provide, it's important to vary your choices throughout the week.

In this chapter you'll find a range of more substantial dishes, any of which are ideally suited to be the center-piece of a dinner or lunch. Choose from a simple stir-fry, an easy one-pot dish or a baked casserole. They're all simple to prepare and accommodate a wide variety of tastes, including beef, pork, lamb, chicken, fish and seafood, as well as delicious vegetarian dishes.

Meat, poultry, fish and eggs

These sources of protein supply essential nutrients such as iron, zinc, and B-vitamins (thiamin, riboflavin, niacin, vitamin B_{12}). But they also contain fat, so it's important to watch serving sizes and use lower-fat cooking methods.

Tips to reduce fat

✿ **Control portion sizes.** A reasonable amount of cooked meat for an adult meal is about 3 oz (75 g) — approximately the size of a deck of cards.

✿ **Choose leaner cuts.** Best bets include round steak, lean ground beef, flank steak, pork tenderloin, chicken and turkey, as well as fish such as haddock, halibut, sole, cod and canned tuna packed in water.

✿ **Cut back on fried or deep-fried meat, fish and poultry.** Try to find lower-fat alternatives to sausages, bacon, hot dogs, deli meats (such as bologna and salami) and regular ground beef.

✿ **Use meat, poultry and fish as complements** to the grains, vegetables, fruit and beans in your meals. For example, the meat portion might account for only one-quarter of your meal.

✿ **Prepare without extra fat or rich sauces.**

Beans, peas, lentils, nuts, seeds and tofu

These sources of vegetable-based protein supply complex carbohydrates and fiber, as well as some B-vitamins (niacin, riboflavin, thiamin and folic acid) and small amounts of minerals such as calcium, iron and potassium. They are generally low in fat, although this is not always the case with tofu and soybeans. Nuts and seeds are typically higher in fat, but their oils provide a source of the antioxidant vitamin E. Because of their fat content, they should be consumed in smaller amounts (for example, 2 to 3 tbsp [25 to 45 mL]).

What about cholesterol?

Meat, poultry, eggs, fish and seafood are a source of dietary cholesterol. Most healthy individuals can enjoy these foods in moderation. Cutting back on fat, especially saturated fat, is the most important strategy for individuals who are concerned about high blood cholesterol.

the challenge *of* VEGETARIAN eating

As a rule, the more foods that are eliminated from the diet, the more challenging it becomes to plan balanced meals. However, a well-planned vegetarian diet that follows *Canada's Food Guide to Healthy Eating* (see pages 176 to 177) and includes plenty of grains, vegetables, dairy products, eggs, fruit, beans, peas, lentils, soy products, nuts and seeds can meet most people's nutritional needs. Nevertheless, some individuals, particularly children and women who are pregnant or breastfeeding, may still have trouble getting the iron, calcium, zinc and vitamin B_{12} they need.

Including eggs and dairy products will increase your intake of calcium and vitamin B_{12}. In fact, vitamin B_{12} is *only* found in animal products such as meat, fish, poultry, eggs, and dairy products. Individuals who avoid these foods will need to consume vitamin B_{12}-fortified products or a B_{12} supplement in order to prevent a nutrient deficiency.

For vegetarians, it is particularly important to eat more foods that are high in iron and calcium. For specific suggestions, see pages 22 and 23.

Cooking to control the fat

Trim all visible fats and skin before cooking. Leave the skin on chicken for cooking, and remove it before eating.

Instead of frying, try baking, roasting, poaching, broiling, grilling or microwaving.

Stir-fry in a nonstick pan using only a small amount of oil or vegetable spray.

WHAT's in a serving?

- One serving of meat, poultry or fish is 50 to 100 g (2 to 3.5 oz) or 1 or 2 eggs.
- One serving of meat alternatives is 1/2 cup to 1 cup (125 to 250 mL) of cooked or canned beans (such as kidney beans, chickpeas, white pea or navy beans) or lentils, 1/3 cup (75 mL) tofu, or 2 tbsp (25 mL) peanut butter.

SERVES 4

Asian Flank Steak

Milutin Ajdacic
TORONTO, ON [P]

Not only is this flank steak a delicious main dish, but it also makes great leftovers! Try it sliced on buns for lunch, added to a vegetable stir-fry or served on top of salad greens with your favorite vinaigrette dressing.

TIP

Marinades that have been exposed to raw meat are contaminated with bacteria. Don't use (as a sauce, for example) unless boiled first.

Complete the meal
Serve
with Quick
Microwave Rice
(see recipe, page 128) and
SAUTÉED SPINACH WITH PINE NUTS
(see recipe, page 99).

1 lb	flank steak	500 g
1/4 cup	soya sauce	50 mL
1/4 cup	granulated sugar	50 mL
2 tbsp	lemon juice	25 mL
1 tbsp	chopped garlic	15 mL
1 tsp	minced ginger	5 mL
1/4 tsp	black pepper	1 mL
1/8 tsp	hot pepper flakes (optional)	0.5 mL

1. Make diagonal slits across top of steak, about 1/8 inch (2 mm) deep. Place in a shallow dish. Set aside.

2. In a bowl combine soya sauce, sugar, lemon juice, garlic, ginger, pepper and, if using, hot pepper flakes. Pour over steak. Marinate, covered, in refrigerator for 4 to 8 hours or overnight, turning a couple of times.

3. Preheat barbecue or broiler. Remove meat from marinade, reserving liquid. Barbecue or grill meat over high heat for 3 to 4 minutes per side or until cooked but still pink in center. Let rest for 5 minutes.

4. Meanwhile, bring reserved marinade to a boil; cook for 5 minutes.

5. Slice meat thinly on the diagonal, across the grain. Drizzle with sauce.

food guide servings

GRAIN PRODUCTS	VEGETABLES & FRUIT
	1
MILK PRODUCTS	MEAT & ALTERNATIVES

nutrient analysis

PER SERVING			
Calories	254	Carbohydrate	15.5 g
Protein	27.2 g	Dietary Fiber	0.2 g
Fat	8.8 g	Sodium	1088 mg

Excellent source of zinc, niacin, vitamin B$_{12}$. **Good** source of iron, vitamin B$_6$.

SERVES   4

Crockpot Beef Stew

Bonnie Conrad, P. Dt.
HALIFAX, NS

In the winter there's nothing more comforting than a plate of hearty beef stew and mashed potatoes.

Make Ahead
Begin cooking this stew early in the day and supper will be ready when you return at night! Stew can be frozen for up to 3 months.

Complete the meal
Serve with mashed potatoes and rolls. Finish the meal with ice cream or frozen yogurt.

1 lb	lean stewing beef, cut into 1-inch (2.5 cm) cubes and patted dry	500 g
1 tbsp	all-purpose flour	15 mL
2 tsp	vegetable oil	10 mL
2 cups	cubed turnips	500 mL
2 cups	cubed carrots	500 mL
1 cup	sliced onions	250 mL
1 1/2 cups	boiling water	375 mL
2	beef bouillon cubes or sachets	2
3 tbsp	red wine vinegar	45 mL
3 tbsp	ketchup	45 mL
4 tsp	prepared mustard	20 mL
1 tsp	Worcestershire sauce	5 mL
2 tbsp	all-purpose flour	25 mL
3 tbsp	cold water	45 mL

1. In a large bowl, toss beef cubes with flour; set aside. In a large nonstick skillet, heat oil over medium-high heat. Add beef and cook for 4 to 5 minutes or until browned on all sides. Place in crockpot. Add turnips, carrots and onions.

2. In a medium bowl, blend together water, bouillon, vinegar, ketchup, mustard and Worcestershire sauce. Add to crockpot; stir gently. Cook, covered, on Low heat setting for 9 hours.

3. In a measuring cup, whisk together flour and water. Add flour mixture to stew; stir gently to blend. Increase crockpot heat setting to High; cook, covered, for 15 minutes or until thickened.

food guide servings

GRAIN PRODUCTS	VEGETABLES & FRUIT
	2 1/2
	1
MILK PRODUCTS	MEAT & ALTERNATIVES

nutrient analysis

PER SERVING			
Calories	308	Carbohydrate	24 g
Protein	28.5 g	Dietary Fiber	4.0 g
Fat	11 g	Sodium	351 mg

Excellent source of iron, zinc, vitamin A, niacin, vitamin B$_6$, vitamin B$_{12}$. **Good** source of vitamin C, riboflavin, folacin. **High** in dietary fiber.

SERVES 8

Fast Chili

Barbara McGillivary
BELLEVILLE, ON   Ⓟ

Food Fast

Try this quick and easy Chili Baked Potato: Scrub a medium (8 oz [250 g]) potato and pierce with a fork; microwave on High for 3 to 4 minutes. Let stand for 2 minutes. Cut an "X" in the top of potato and squeeze open. Top with hot chili and shredded cheese.

Nutrition Facts

This chili provides an incredible 18 g fiber per serving. That's more than most Canadians eat in a whole day! When introducing more fiber into your diet, remember to drink plenty of fluids to help with proper digestion.

Make Ahead

Double the ingredients in this recipe to make an extra batch. If planning to freeze, use fresh (not previously frozen) ground beef. Freeze extra chili in airtight containers in portion sizes suited to your needs. Keep for up to 3 months in the freezer.

1 lb	lean ground beef	500 g
1	can (19 oz [540 mL]) stewed tomatoes	1
2	cans (each 14 oz [398 mL]) beans in tomato sauce	2
2	cans (each 19 oz [540 mL]) kidney beans, rinsed and drained	2
1 cup	sliced white or red onions	250 mL
2 cups	diced green bell peppers	500 mL
1 tbsp	chili powder	15 mL

1. In a large saucepan or Dutch oven over medium-high heat, brown meat until no longer pink inside. Drain fat.

2. Add tomatoes, beans in tomato sauce, kidney beans, onions, green peppers and chili powder. Reduce heat and simmer, covered and stirring occasionally, for 20 to 30 minutes.

Complete the meal

Serve with whole-wheat toast or CORNMEAL MUFFINS (see recipe, page 34) and a tossed green salad or vegetable sticks. Cool your palate with lemon or lime sherbet.

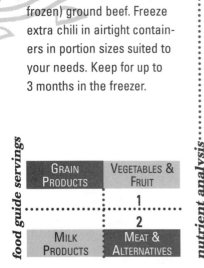

food guide servings

GRAIN PRODUCTS	VEGETABLES & FRUIT
	1
	2
MILK PRODUCTS	MEAT & ALTERNATIVES

nutrient analysis

PER SERVING			
Calories	338	Carbohydrate	50.3 g
Protein	24.4 g	Dietary Fiber	18.0 g
Fat	6.5 g	Sodium	958 mg

Excellent source of vitamin C, thiamin, niacin, folacin, vitamin B_{12}, zinc. **Good** source of riboflavin, vitamin B_6, iron. **Very high** in dietary fiber.

SERVES 4 Hoisin Beef and Broccoli Stir-Fry

Bev Callaghan, RD

2 tsp	vegetable oil	10 mL
12 oz	sirloin or inside round steak, cut into 3- by 1/2-inch (7.5 by 1 cm) strips	375 g
1 tbsp	chopped ginger root	15 mL
1 tsp	minced garlic	5 mL
3 cups	small broccoli florets	750 mL
1/3 cup	sliced water chestnuts	75 mL
1/2 tsp	cornstarch	2 mL
1/3 cup	orange juice *or* beef stock	75 mL
2 tbsp	hoisin sauce	25 mL
1/2 tsp	sesame oil (optional)	2 mL
	Black pepper	
1 tbsp	toasted sesame seeds (optional)	15 mL

1. In a large nonstick skillet, heat oil over medium-high heat; add beef strips and stir-fry for 1 to 2 minutes or until browned. Add ginger, garlic, broccoli and water chestnuts; stir-fry for another 2 to 3 minutes or until broccoli is tender-crisp.

2. In a small bowl or glass measuring cup, whisk together cornstarch, orange juice, hoisin sauce and, if using, sesame oil. Add to skillet; cook, stirring, for 1 to 2 minutes or until thickened and heated through. Season to taste with pepper. Serve over rice. If desired, sprinkle with sesame seeds.

GRAIN PRODUCTS	VEGETABLES & FRUIT
	1
	1
MILK PRODUCTS	MEAT & ALTERNATIVES

nutrient analysis

PER SERVING			
Calories	178	Carbohydrate	11.0 g
Protein	19.9 g	Dietary Fiber	1.6 g
Fat	6.0 g	Sodium	195 mg

Excellent source of vitamin C, niacin, vitamin B_{12}, zinc. **Good** source of riboflavin, vitamin B_6, iron.

SERVES 8

Lazy Lasagna

Bev Callaghan RD
Lynn Roblin RD   [P]

PREHEAT OVEN TO 350° F (180° C)
13- BY 9-INCH (3 L) BAKING DISH, GREASED

Here's a quick way to get all the satisfying flavor and texture of lasagna without spending a lot of time in the kitchen. It's a perfect lunch-box treat – just heat it up in the microwave in the morning, pop into a short, wide-mouth thermos, pack with the rest of your lunch and off you go.

Make Ahead
When you have time to cook, bake up two batches of this lasagna. Enjoy one batch for supper then divide the other into individual portions, freeze in airtight containers and use as needed for meals or lunches. If planning to freeze, use fresh (not previously frozen) ground beef.

Complete the meal
This is a fabulous four-food-group recipe. If you wish, serve it with a green salad and low-fat salad dressing.

3 cups	penne, rotini or other large pasta	750 mL
2 tsp	olive oil	10 mL
12 oz	lean ground beef	375 g
1/2 cup	chopped onions	125 mL
1 cup	finely chopped or grated carrots	250 mL
1	jar (24 to 25 oz [700 to 750 mL]) prepared tomato pasta sauce	1
1/2 tsp	Italian seasoning *or* dried oregano *or* basil	2 mL
1	container (17 oz [475 g]) light ricotta cheese	1
1	egg	1
1 1/2 cups	grated partly skimmed mozzarella cheese	375 mL
1/4 cup	grated Parmesan cheese	50 mL

1. In a large pot of boiling water, cook pasta until tender but firm; drain. Toss with olive oil; set aside.

2. In a large skillet, cook beef over medium-high heat until browned. Add onions and carrots; cook for 3 to 4 minutes. Stir in pasta sauce and Italian seasoning. Remove from heat and set aside.

3. In a bowl combine ricotta cheese, egg and 1 cup (250 mL) of the mozzarella cheese. Set aside.

4. To assemble: Spread half of the meat mixture on bottom of baking dish. Top with all of the pasta. Spread all of the cheese mixture over pasta. Top with remaining meat mixture. Sprinkle with remaining 1/2 cup (125 mL) mozzarella cheese and Parmesan cheese.

5. Bake in preheated oven, uncovered, for 35 to 45 minutes or until bubbling and brown on top. Let stand for 10 minutes before serving.

food guide servings

GRAIN PRODUCTS	VEGETABLES & FRUIT
1	1
1	1/2
MILK PRODUCTS	MEAT & ALTERNATIVES

nutrient analysis

PER SERVING			
Calories	461	Carbohydrate	43.9 g
Protein	28.4 g	Dietary Fiber	3.6 g
Fat	18.9 g	Sodium	747 mg

Excellent source of vitamin A, riboflavin, niacin, vitamin B$_6$, folacin, vitamin B$_{12}$, calcium, zinc. **Good** source of thiamin, iron. **Moderate** source of dietary fiber.

Meatloaf "Muffins" with Barbecue Sauce

Diana Callaghan
RICHARD'S LANDING, ON [P]

PREHEAT OVEN TO 375° F (190° C)
12-CUP MUFFIN TIN, GREASED

Meatloaf "Muffins"

1 1/2 lbs	lean ground beef	750 g
3/4 cup	oatmeal *or* dry bread crumbs *or* cracker crumbs	175 mL
1/4 cup	wheat bran	50 mL
1	can (5.4 oz [160 mL]) evaporated 2% milk	1
1	egg	1
1 tsp	chili powder	5 mL
1/2 tsp	garlic powder	2 mL
1/4 tsp	salt	1 mL
1/4 tsp	black pepper	1 mL

Barbecue Sauce

1 cup	ketchup	250 mL
1/4 cup	finely chopped onion	50 mL
2 tbsp	brown sugar	25 mL
1/2 tsp	hot pepper sauce (optional)	2 mL

1. Muffins: In a large bowl, combine ground beef, oatmeal, bran, milk, egg, chili powder, garlic powder, salt and pepper. Divide mixture evenly among muffin cups, pressing down lightly.

2. Sauce: In another bowl, combine ketchup, onion, sugar and, if using, hot pepper sauce. Spoon about 1 tbsp (15 mL) sauce over each muffin.

3. Bake in preheated oven for 25 to 30 minutes or until meat is no longer pink in center.

GRAIN PRODUCTS	VEGETABLES & FRUIT
1/2	1/2
1/4	1
MILK PRODUCTS	MEAT & ALTERNATIVES

nutrient analysis

PER SERVING		
Calories	396	Carbohydrate 29.4 g
Protein	27.2 g	Dietary Fiber 3.2 g
Fat	19.5 g	Sodium 757 mg

Excellent source of niacin, vitamin B_{12}, iron, zinc. **Good** source of riboflavin, vitamin B_6. **Moderate** source of dietary fiber.

SERVES 6

Patricia Cissell, RD
MISSISSAUGA, ON

 P

Pastitsio

PREHEAT OVEN TO 350° F (180° C)
10-CUP (2.5 L) DEEP BAKING DISH, GREASED

This Greek pasta dish is started in the microwave to save time, then baked to perfection in the oven.

Make Ahead

Prepare this recipe to the end of Step 3 up to one day ahead. Keep refrigerated, then proceed with remaining steps in recipe. Increase baking time by 5 to 10 minutes.

Nutrition Facts

Use lower-fat salad dressings to complement higher-fat meals (containing less than 3 g fat per 1 tbsp [15 mL] serving).

1 1/2 cups	macaroni	375 mL
1 lb	lean ground beef	500 g
1/2 cup	chopped onions	125 mL
1/2 cup	chopped celery	125 mL
1/2 tsp	minced garlic	2 mL
1 cup	tomato sauce	250 mL
3/4 tsp	salt	7 mL
1/2 tsp	cinnamon	2 mL
1/4 tsp	dried oregano	1 mL
1/8 tsp	black pepper	0.5 mL
1/2 cup	grated Parmesan cheese	125 mL

White Sauce

2 tbsp	butter *or* margarine	25 mL
3 tbsp	flour	45 mL
1 1/2 cups	milk	375 mL
1	egg, beaten	1

1. In a large pot of boiling water, cook pasta according to package directions or until tender but firm; drain. Set aside.

2. In a large microwave-safe bowl, crumble ground beef. Stir in onions, celery and garlic. Microwave on High, stirring at 2-minute intervals, for 5 to 6 minutes or until beef is no longer pink. Drain fat. Stir in tomato sauce, 1/2 tsp (2 mL) of the salt, cinnamon, oregano and pepper. Set aside.

3. Place half the macaroni in baking dish; sprinkle with 1/4 cup (50 mL) Parmesan cheese. Spread meat mixture evenly over macaroni; top with remaining macaroni.

4. White Sauce: In a microwave-safe bowl, melt butter on Medium for 1 minute; stir in flour and remaining salt. Gradually whisk in milk until mixture is smooth. Microwave on Medium, stirring at 2-minute intervals, for 5 to 6 minutes or until thickened.

5. In a small bowl, quickly stir a small amount of sauce into egg. Stir egg mixture into white sauce. Add remaining Parmesan cheese; blend well. Pour over macaroni; insert knife into mixture in several places so sauce can penetrate layers. Bake in pre-heated oven for 30 to 40 minutes or until top is golden and casserole is set. Let stand for 5 minutes before serving.

Complete the meal

Serve with a crisp salad and Greek-style vinaigrette salad dressing.

food guide servings

Grain Products	Vegetables & Fruit
1	1/2
1/2	1
Milk Products	Meat & Alternatives

nutrient analysis

PER SERVING			
Calories	361	Carbohydrate	30.7 g
Protein	24.6 g	Dietary Fiber	2.2 g
Fat	15.2 g	Sodium	806 mg

Excellent source of zinc, riboflavin, niacin, folacin, vitamin B_{12}. **Good** source of calcium, iron, thiamin, vitamin B_6. **Moderate** source of dietary fiber.

SERVES 6

*Lynn Homer RD
Meals on Wheels*
CALGARY, AB

This recipe comes from the Calgary Meals on Wheels program, and makes a wonderful meal to share with good friends and family. Be sure to have plenty of mashed potatoes to enjoy with the savory gravy.

TIP

To tenderize steaks, place meat between 2 pieces of plastic wrap and pound with a flat wooden or rubber mallet until flattened slightly. (The heel of a wine bottle also works well!) This process helps to break down the tough fibers in the meat.

Make Ahead

This recipe can be prepared to the end of Step 3, up to 1 day ahead. Refrigerate until ready to cook and increase baking time by 10 minutes.

Salisbury Steak in Wine Sauce

PREHEAT OVEN TO 350° F (180° C)
11- BY 7-INCH (2 L) BAKING DISH, GREASED

2 tbsp	vegetable oil	25 mL
6	4-oz (125 g) tenderized round steaks, (see Tip, at left), pounded to 1/2-inch (1 cm) thickness and patted dry	6
1 cup	sliced onions	250 mL
2 cups	sliced mushrooms	500 mL
3 tbsp	flour	45 mL
1	beef bouillon cube	1
1 1/2 cups	hot water	375 mL
1/2 cup	dry red wine	125 mL
2 tsp	Worcestershire sauce	10 mL
1/2 tsp	garlic powder	2 mL
1/2 tsp	paprika	2 mL
1	bay leaf	1
1/8 tsp	black pepper	0.5 mL
1 tbsp	chopped fresh parsley (optional)	15 mL

1. In a large nonstick skillet, heat 1 tsp (5 mL) of the oil over medium-high heat. Cook steaks in 2 batches, turning once, until brown on both sides. Transfer steaks to prepared baking dish when cooked.

2. Heat another 1 tsp (5 mL) of the oil in skillet. Add onions and mushrooms; cook for 5 to 6 minutes or until softened. Transfer to baking dish, placing vegetables on top of steaks. Remove skillet from heat and add remaining oil; blend in flour.

3. In a small bowl, dissolve bouillon cube in hot water. Slowly add bouillon to flour mixture, whisking constantly until well combined. Return skillet to medium heat; stir in wine, Worcestershire sauce, garlic powder, paprika, bay leaf and pepper. Continue to whisk constantly for 3 to 4 minutes or until sauce is thickened and smooth. Pour sauce over steaks.

4. Bake, covered, for 45 to 50 minutes or until meat is fork-tender. Remove bay leaf before serving. Sprinkle with parsley, if desired.

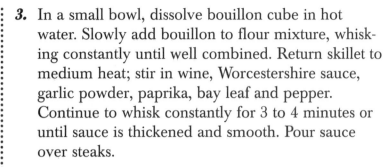

Complete the meal

Serve with mashed potatoes and frozen green peas. Finish the meal with Lunchbox Applesauce Cake *(see recipe, page 166).*

nutrient analysis

GRAIN PRODUCTS	VEGETABLES & FRUIT
	1/2
	1
MILK PRODUCTS	MEAT & ALTERNATIVES

PER SERVING			
Calories	212	Carbohydrate	7.2 g
Protein	27.7 g	Dietary Fiber	0.9 g
Fat	7.2 g	Sodium	242 mg

Excellent source of niacin, vitamin B$_6$, vitamin B$_{12}$, zinc. **Good** source of riboflavin, iron.

SERVES 6 Veggie, Beef and Pasta Bake

Kathryn Papple
Brant County Health Unit **P**
BRANTFORD, ON

Here's a terrific recipe that makes a complete meal, with something from all 4 food groups! The pasta does not require any pre-cooking so you save preparation and clean-up time.

TIP

If you are concerned about sodium, use light soya sauce instead of the regular variety. One tbsp (15 mL) regular soya sauce contains 1037 mg sodium; the same amount of sodium-reduced or light soya sauce contains only 605 mg.

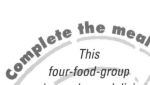

Complete the meal

This four-food-group recipe makes a delicious complete meal. But crusty bread makes a great accompaniment.

PREHEAT OVEN TO 350° F (180° C)
13- BY 9-INCH (3 L) BAKING DISH, GREASED

1 lb	lean ground beef	500 g
1 cup	sliced onions	250 mL
1 cup	diced zucchini	250 mL
2 tsp	minced garlic	10 mL
1	can (28 oz [796 mL]) stewed or diced tomatoes, with juice	1
2 tbsp	sodium-reduced soya sauce	25 mL
1/2 tsp	crushed red pepper flakes	2 mL
2 cups	rotini (or other spiral pasta)	500 mL
1 1/2 cups	shredded Cheddar cheese	375 mL

1. In a large nonstick skillet over medium-high heat, combine ground beef, onions, zucchini and garlic; cook for 8 to 10 minutes or until beef is no longer pink and vegetables are softened. Drain fat; pour beef mixture into baking dish. Set aside.

2. Meanwhile, drain juice from tomatoes into an 8-cup (2 L) microwave-safe measuring cup; add water to make 2 cups (500 mL). Roughly chop tomatoes; add to measuring cup. Stir in soya sauce and red pepper flakes. Microwave on High for 5 minutes or until very hot. Stir in rotini.

3. Pour tomato-pasta mixture into baking dish and combine with meat mixture. Press pasta down to make sure it is submerged in the liquid. Bake in preheated oven, covered, for 20 minutes. Remove cover; stir gently and sprinkle with cheese. Bake, uncovered, for 15 to 20 minutes or until pasta is tender.

food guide servings

GRAIN PRODUCTS	VEGETABLES & FRUIT
1/2	1 1/2
1/2	1
MILK PRODUCTS	MEAT & ALTERNATIVES

nutrient analysis

PER SERVING			
Calories	352	Carbohydrate	26.1 g
Protein	25.1 g	Dietary Fiber	3.0 g
Fat	16.8 g	Sodium	778 mg

Excellent source of iron, zinc, riboflavin, niacin, folacin, vitamin B_{12}. **Good** source of calcium, vitamin A, vitamin C, thiamin, vitamin B_6. **Moderate** source of dietary fiber.

SERVES 4

Bev Callaghan, RD

Broiled Ham Steak with Pineapple-Mango Salsa

PREHEAT BROILER
SHALLOW BAKING DISH, GREASED

The Pineapple-Mango Salsa in this recipe is also great with grilled salmon or swordfish. For lunch, try it stuffed in a pita with chicken salad or rolled up in a tortilla with light cream cheese and some thinly sliced ham or smoked turkey.

2	6-oz (175 g) packaged ham steaks	2
2 tsp	Dijon or other mustard	10 mL
2 tsp	brown sugar	10 mL
1 tbsp	orange juice *or* pineapple juice	15 mL

Pineapple-Mango Salsa

1 cup	diced fresh mango	250 mL
1 cup	diced fresh pineapple	250 mL
1/2 cup	chopped red onions	125 mL
1/4 cup	finely chopped cilantro	50 mL
2 tbsp	lime juice	25 mL

TIP

Fresh pineapple tastes best in this recipe, but you can use canned pineapple instead.

Choose a ripe mango that is red or orange-yellow and soft to the touch.

Make Ahead

The salsa can be made ahead and kept in the refrigerator for several days.

Nutrition Facts

Ham, bacon and many processed deli meats are often high in salt. If you are concerned about excess sodium, you may need to limit your consumption of these foods.

1. Place ham steaks in baking dish and spread with mustard. Sprinkle with brown sugar, then orange juice. Broil for 2 to 3 minutes or until golden and bubbling.

2. Pineapple-Mango Salsa: In a bowl stir together mango, pineapple, onions, cilantro and lime juice. Chill until ready to use. Warm to room temperature before serving with ham steak.

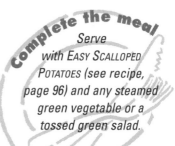

Complete the meal

Serve with EASY SCALLOPED POTATOES (see recipe, page 96) and any steamed green vegetable or a tossed green salad.

GRAIN PRODUCTS	VEGETABLES & FRUIT
	1
	1
MILK PRODUCTS	MEAT & ALTERNATIVES

nutrient analysis

PER SERVING			
Calories	175	Carbohydrate	17.0 g
Protein	18.0 g	Dietary Fiber	1.7 g
Fat	4.2 g	Sodium	1148 mg

Excellent source of thiamin, niacin. **Good** source of vitamin A, vitamin C, vitamin B_6, vitamin B_{12}, zinc.

SERVES 6

Bev Callaghan, RD

Barbecued Butterflied Leg of Lamb

Here we use a Greek-style marinade. It's the perfect companion to grilled lamb, which is best served medium-rare.

Nutrition Facts

Watch your meat consumption and you'll be well on your way to controlling your fat intake. A serving of meat should be about the size of the palm of your hand.

1	2-lb (1 kg) butterflied leg of lamb, trimmed	1
1 tsp	minced garlic	5 mL
2 tbsp	lemon juice	25 mL
2 tbsp	chopped fresh oregano (or 2 tsp [10 mL] dried)	25 mL
2 tbsp	chopped fresh mint (or 2 tsp [10 mL] dried)	25 mL
1 tbsp	olive oil	15 mL
	Black pepper	

1. Place lamb in a large shallow dish, fat-side down. Spread with garlic. Sprinkle with lemon juice, oregano, mint and olive oil. Season to taste with pepper.

2. Cover and marinate in the refrigerator, turning once or twice, for 2 hours or overnight. Remove from fridge 30 minutes before grilling.

3. Preheat barbecue or broiler. For medium-rare, barbecue on greased grill for 10 to 12 minutes per side, depending on thickness of lamb or, if using a meat thermometer, until the internal temperature of lamb registers 140 to 150° F (60 to 65° C).

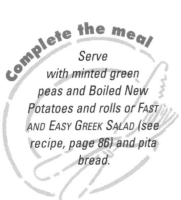

Complete the meal

Serve with minted green peas and Boiled New Potatoes and rolls or FAST AND EASY GREEK SALAD (see recipe, page 86) and pita bread.

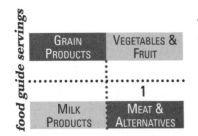

food guide servings

GRAIN PRODUCTS	VEGETABLES & FRUIT
	1
MILK PRODUCTS	MEAT & ALTERNATIVES

nutrient analysis

PER SERVING			
Calories	177	Carbohydrate	0.7 g
Protein	26.3 g	Dietary Fiber	0.1 g
Fat	7.0 g	Sodium	44 mg

Excellent source of zinc, riboflavin, niacin, vitamin B$_{12}$. **Good** source of iron.

Bev Callaghan, RD

SERVES 4

Grilled Lamb Chops with Sautéed Peppers and Zucchini

Try this impressive dish for your next dinner party. Your guests need never know how easy it is to make!

TIP

For extra-easy clean up, line the broiler pan with foil.

If weather permits, grill chops on the barbecue; you'll improve their flavor – and enjoy some time outdoors!

To cook the vegetables on the grill, place vegetables and sauce in a heavy-duty foil packet and barbecue for about 10 minutes, turning once.

Complete the meal

Serve with couscous or rice. For the perfect finish to a special occasion, serve ORANGE CRÈME CARAMEL (see recipe, page 168) for dessert.

PREHEAT BROILER OR BARBECUE

1/4 cup	balsamic or red wine vinegar	50 mL
2 tbsp	olive oil	25 mL
1 tbsp	Dijon mustard	15 mL
1 tsp	dried thyme leaves	5 mL
1 tsp	minced garlic	5 mL
1/8 tsp	black pepper	0.5 mL
8 to 12	bone-in, center-cut loin lamb chops, trimmed of fat (about 1 1/2 lbs [750 g] in total)	8 to 12
1 1/2 cups	sliced zucchini	375 mL
1 1/2 cups	julienned red bell peppers	375 mL
1 cup	sliced sweet onions	250 mL

1. In a large bowl, blend together vinegar, 1 tbsp (15 mL) of the oil, mustard, thyme, garlic and pepper. Transfer 2 to 3 tbsp (25 to 45 mL) of the mixture to a small bowl; set aside.

2. Place chops on broiling pan; spoon reserved vinaigrette on top. Grill under broiler, turning once, for 8 to 10 minutes or until cooked to desired doneness.

3. Meanwhile, in a large nonstick skillet, heat remaining 1 tbsp (15 mL) oil over medium-high heat. Add zucchini, peppers and onions; stir-fry for 6 to 8 minutes or until tender-crisp. Add remaining vinaigrette to pan; cook, stirring, for 1 to 2 minutes or until heated through.

GRAIN PRODUCTS	VEGETABLES & FRUIT
	2
	1
MILK PRODUCTS	MEAT & ALTERNATIVES

nutrient analysis

PER SERVING			
Calories	233	Carbohydrate	12.2 g
Protein	19.0 g	Dietary Fiber	1.9 g
Fat	12.2 g	Sodium	87 mg

Excellent source of vitamin C, niacin, vitamin B$_{12}$. **Good** source of iron, zinc, vitamin A, riboflavin.

SERVES 4 Polynesian Pork Kebabs

Bev Callaghan, RD

EIGHT 8-INCH (20 CM) WOODEN SKEWERS

These colorful kebabs are perfect for casual entertaining or for a special family meal.

TIP
Soak wooden skewers for 30 minutes to prevent them from burning on the barbecue.

To prevent bacterial contamination, use a clean platter to bring kebabs back into the house.

Fresh pineapple works best in this recipe; it has a firmer texture and, unlike canned pineapple, can be cut into larger chunks.

Quick Couscous
Place 1 cup (250 mL) couscous in a medium ovenproof bowl with a dash of olive oil. Pour 1 cup (250 mL) boiling water on top of couscous; stir. Cover and let stand for 5 minutes. Fluff with a fork. Makes 3 cups (750 mL). One half cup (125 mL) couscous provides 1 Grain Products serving.

1/4 cup	sodium-reduced soya sauce	50 mL
2 tbsp	lemon juice	25 mL
2 tbsp	liquid honey *or* brown sugar	25 mL
1 tsp	vegetable oil	5 mL
1 tsp	ground ginger *or* 1/2 tsp (2 mL) minced ginger root	5 mL
1 lb	lean pork loin or tenderloin, cubed	500 g
1 1/2 cups	cubed fresh pineapple	375 mL
1	red bell pepper, cut into chunks	1
1	green bell pepper, cut into chunks	1

1. In a medium bowl, combine soya sauce, lemon juice, honey, oil and ginger; add pork cubes, tossing to coat. Cover and marinate for at least 30 minutes or overnight in refrigerator.

2. Thread skewers alternately with pieces of pork, pineapple, red pepper and green pepper. Brush kebabs with marinade; discard any left over.

3. Preheat barbecue or broiler. Barbecue kebabs over medium-high heat, turning once, for 10 to 12 minutes or until pork is just slightly pink in the center. Alternatively, grill under broiler, turning once, for 8 to 10 minutes or until cooked through.

complete the meal
Serve these kebabs on a bed of couscous. For dessert, try COUNTRY APPLE BERRY CRISP (see recipe, page 162).

food guide servings

GRAIN PRODUCTS	VEGETABLES & FRUIT
	2
	1
MILK PRODUCTS	MEAT & ALTERNATIVES

nutrient analysis

PER SERVING			
Calories	235	Carbohydrate	16.5 g
Protein	26.7 g	Dietary Fiber	1.6 g
Fat	7.0 g	Sodium	362 mg

Excellent source of vitamin C, thiamin, niacin, vitamin B_6, vitamin B_{12}. **Good** source of riboflavin, iron.

Pork Chops with Peaches and Kiwi

Johanne Thériault, RD
MONCTON, NB   [P]

SERVES 4

TIP

Instead of fresh peaches, you can use 1 can (14 oz [398 mL]) drained sliced peaches or use nectarines or mangoes.

Young children often prefer fruit "straight up" – that is, without sauce. In this case, prepare extra fruit and serve it alone as a side dish.

Food Fast

If you are serving this dish with rice, start cooking it while you prepare the rest of the meal.

Nutrition Facts

Experiment with new ways to include more fruit in your main meals. Dark orange fruit like peaches, mangoes and nectarines provide vitamins A and C, as well as some fiber.

Complete the meal

Serve with Quick Microwave Rice (see page 128) or noodles. Have pudding and CRANBERRY OATMEAL COOKIES (see recipe, page 160) for dessert.

3/4 cup	chicken stock	175 mL
1/2 cup	orange juice	125 mL
4 tsp	cornstarch	20 mL
2 tsp	granulated sugar	10 mL
1 tsp	minced garlic	5 mL
1 tsp	minced ginger root (or 1/4 tsp [1 mL] ground ginger)	5 mL
1/2 tsp	grated lemon zest (optional)	2 mL
1 tsp	olive oil	5 mL
4	lean boneless or bone-in pork chops	4
1 1/2 cups	sliced peaches	375 mL
1/2 cup	sliced (cut lengthwise) peeled kiwi fruit	125 mL
	Salt	
	Black pepper	

1. In a medium bowl, combine stock, orange juice, cornstarch, sugar, garlic, ginger and lemon zest. Set aside.

2. In a large nonstick skillet, heat oil over medium-high heat. Add pork chops and sear for 1 to 2 minutes per side or until golden. Add stock mixture; bring to a boil. Reduce heat to medium-low and simmer for 5 to 6 minutes or until pork is cooked and just slightly pink at the center. Stir in peaches and kiwi. Season to taste with salt and pepper. Simmer for 1 to 2 minutes or until heated through.

GRAIN PRODUCTS	VEGETABLES & FRUIT
	1
	1
MILK PRODUCTS	MEAT & ALTERNATIVES

nutrient analysis

PER SERVING			
Calories	234	Carbohydrate	18.7 g
Protein	23.3 g	Dietary Fiber	1.7 g
Fat	7.2 g	Sodium	209 mg

Excellent source of zinc, thiamin, niacin, vitamin B_{12}. **Good** source of vitamin C, riboflavin, vitamin B_6.

SERVES 3

Bev Callaghan, RD

Pork Tenderloin with Roasted Potatoes

PREHEAT OVEN TO 375° F (190° C)
11- BY 7-INCH (2 L) BAKING DISH, GREASED

This dish takes only 10 minutes to prepare. And because it cooks in one baking dish, clean-up is a snap!

TIP

If you need to feed more than 3 people, just buy another pork tenderloin and double up the remaining ingredients. If you have leftovers, add slices of tenderloin to EGG AND MUSHROOM FRIED RICE (see recipe, page 54) or use in sandwiches.

Nutrition Facts

Instead of greasing pans and adding more fat to your meals, use a small amount of vegetable oil spray.

To boost your beta carotene intake, replace 1 cup (250 mL) white potatoes with sweet potatoes.

1	12-oz (375 g) pork tenderloin	1
2 tsp	orange marmalade	10 mL
2 tsp	Dijon mustard	10 mL
1 tsp	vegetable oil	5 mL
2 cups	potatoes, cut into 1-inch (2.5 cm) pieces	500 mL
1 tbsp	lemon juice	15 ml
1 tsp	crumbled dried rosemary	5 mL

1. Pat pork tenderloin dry; place in center of baking dish.

2. In a small bowl, combine marmalade, mustard and 1/2 tsp (2 mL) of the oil; brush over pork.

3. In a medium bowl, toss potatoes with remaining oil; arrange around pork in baking dish. Sprinkle potatoes with lemon juice. Sprinkle pork and potatoes with rosemary. Bake in preheated oven for 40 to 45 minutes or until pork is just slightly pink at center and potatoes are tender. Cut pork into 1/2-inch (1 cm) slices before serving.

Complete the meal

Serve with green beans, applesauce and whole-grain rolls and a glass of milk.

food guide servings

GRAIN PRODUCTS	VEGETABLES & FRUIT
	1
	1
MILK PRODUCTS	MEAT & ALTERNATIVES

nutrient analysis

PER SERVING			
Calories	236	Carbohydrate	17.5 g
Protein	29.3 g	Dietary Fiber	1.6 g
Fat	5.1 g	Sodium	103 mg

Excellent source of thiamin, niacin, vitamin B_6, vitamin B_{12}, zinc.
Good source of riboflavin, iron.

Skillet Pork Chops with Sweet Potatoes and Couscous

SERVES 4

Bev Callaghan, RD P

This "meal in a skillet" is the perfect solution for a busy weeknight supper.

TIP

You can substitute 1 cup (250 mL) chicken stock for the bouillon cube and water.

Nutrition Facts
When you focus your meals around grains and vegetables, you'll be sure to keep your fat intake under control.

Whenever possible, choose nutrient-rich vegetables that are dark orange, red or green in color.

Complete the meal
Balance this dish with something from the Milk Products food group.

2 tsp	vegetable oil	10 mL
4	boneless pork loin chops, trimmed and patted dry (about 1 lb [500 g])	4
1/2 cup	chopped onions	125 mL
1/2 cup	chopped celery or fennel	125 mL
2 cups	diced sweet potatoes	500 mL
1	chicken bouillon cube dissolved in 1 cup (250 mL) water	1
1/2 to 1 tsp	crumbled dried rosemary	2 to 5 mL
3/4 cup	orange juice *or* apple juice	175 mL
1 cup	quick-cooking couscous	250 mL
	Black pepper	

1. In a large nonstick skillet, heat 1 tsp (5 mL) of the oil over medium-high heat. Add pork chops and cook, turning once, for 7 to 8 minutes or until slightly pink at center and juices run clear when pierced with a fork. Transfer pork to a plate and keep warm.

2. Add remaining oil to skillet. Add onions and celery; cook for 3 minutes. Add sweet potatoes, bouillon mixture and rosemary; bring to a boil. Reduce heat and simmer, covered, for 7 to 8 minutes or until potatoes are barely tender.

3. Stir in orange juice and couscous. Return pork to skillet and simmer, covered, for 2 minutes. Remove pan from heat and let stand for 3 minutes. Fluff couscous with fork. Season to taste with pepper.

GRAIN PRODUCTS	VEGETABLES & FRUIT
1 1/2	1 1/2
	1
MILK PRODUCTS	MEAT & ALTERNATIVES

nutrient analysis

PER SERVING			
Calories	462	Carbohydrate	59.6 g
Protein	32.7 g	Dietary Fiber	4.3 g
Fat	9.4 g	Sodium	397 mg

Excellent source of zinc, vitamin A, thiamin, niacin, vitamin B6, vitamin B12. **Good** source of vitamin C, riboflavin, folacin. **High** in dietary fiber.

SERVES 4

Gabriella Barna-Adorjan
Toronto, ON   P

Gabriella uses Hungarian paprika from the city of Szeged which is available from Hungarian and fine food delicatessens.

TIP

Need to feed a crowd? Just double this family-friendly recipe and use 2 baking dishes.

For a nice color contrast, use a mixture of red and green bell peppers.

This meal makes yummy leftovers; just make sure you enjoy them within 3 days. For more information on how long to keep leftovers, check out the chart "How Long Will it Keep?" (see page 174).

Baked Chicken and Potato Dinner

PREHEAT OVEN TO 400° F (200° C)
13- BY 9-INCH (3 L) BAKING DISH

4	skinless bone-in chicken breasts	4
2	medium unpeeled russet potatoes, cut into 1-inch (2.5 cm) cubes	2
1 cup	green and/or red bell peppers, cut into 1-inch (2.5 cm) cubes	250 mL
1	medium onion, cut into 8 pieces	1
2 tbsp	olive oil	25 mL
1 tsp	garlic powder	5 mL
1 tsp	Hungarian paprika	5 mL
1/4 cup	grated Parmesan cheese	50 mL

1. Pat chicken breasts dry with paper towel; place one breast in each corner of baking dish. Put potatoes, peppers and onion in center of dish. Drizzle olive oil over chicken and vegetables; sprinkle with garlic powder, paprika and cheese.

2. Bake in preheated oven, stirring vegetables once halfway through cooking time, for 40 to 50 minutes or until juices run clear when chicken is pierced with a fork and vegetables are tender.

complete the meal

Serve with HONEY-GLAZED CARROTS (see recipe, page 97), or green beans and whole-grain rolls.

food guide servings

GRAIN PRODUCTS	VEGETABLES & FRUIT
	2 1/2
1/4	1
MILK PRODUCTS	MEAT & ALTERNATIVES

nutrient analysis

PER SERVING			
Calories	387	Carbohydrate	33.4 g
Protein	37.8 g	Dietary Fiber	3.4 g
Fat	11.0 g	Sodium	199 mg

Excellent source of vitamin C, niacin, vitamin B_6. **Good** source of thiamin, vitamin B_{12}, iron, zinc. **Moderate** source of dietary fiber.

SERVES 4 Baked Chicken Parmesan

Beth Callaghan, RD

P

PREHEAT OVEN TO 350° F (180° C)
11- BY 7-INCH (2 L) BAKING DISH, GREASED

If you use a commercially prepared pasta sauce in this recipe, remember that it will increase your sodium intake.

TIP

After preparing uncooked meat and poultry, be sure to clean cutting boards and utensils in hot soapy water and sanitize by rinsing in hot water that has a capful of bleach added to it. Having two cutting boards – one for raw meat and the other for everything else – helps reduce chances of bacterial contamination.

Complete the meal

Add some rice or pasta and this dish becomes a complete meal.

2 tsp	vegetable oil	10 mL
4	boneless skinless chicken breasts	4
1 cup	diced zucchini	250 mL
1/2 cup	sliced onions	125mL
1 1/2 cups	PIQUANT TOMATO SAUCE (see recipe, page 150) *or* commercially prepared tomato pasta sauce	375 mL
1 tsp	dried basil *or* Italian seasoning	5 mL
1 cup	grated partly skimmed mozzarella cheese	250 mL
1/2 cup	Parmesan cheese	125 mL

1. In a large nonstick skillet, heat 1 tsp (5 mL) of the oil over medium-high heat. Add chicken breasts and sear for 1 to 2 minutes per side or until golden brown. Transfer to baking dish.

2. Heat remaining oil in skillet. Add zucchini and onions; sauté for 3 to 5 minutes or until lightly browned. Remove from pan and place on top of chicken.

3. In a small bowl, blend together PIQUANT TOMATO SAUCE and basil; pour over chicken and vegetables. Sprinkle with mozzarella and Parmesan cheese. Bake in preheated oven for 25 to 30 minutes or until juices run clear when chicken is pierced with a fork.

GRAIN PRODUCTS	VEGETABLES & FRUIT
	2
1	1
MILK PRODUCTS	MEAT & ALTERNATIVES

nutrient analysis

PER SERVING			
Calories	372	Carbohydrate	12.0 g
Protein	47.0 g	Dietary Fiber	2.4 g
Fat	14.7 g	Sodium	542 mg

Excellent source of calcium, zinc, niacin, vitamin B_6, vitamin B_{12}. **Good** source of vitamin A, riboflavin. **Moderate** source of dietary fiber.

SERVES 4 Chinese Almond Chicken with Noodles

Stephanie Buckle, RD
CORNER BROOK, NF

When she makes this recipe, Stephanie saves time by using bouillon cubes and water to make chicken stock. For less salt, try using a sodium-reduced type of bouillon cube.

TIP

To toast almonds: In a non-stick skillet over medium heat, toast almonds, stirring constantly, for 3 to 4 minutes or until golden brown. Alternatively, microwave on High for 3 to 5 minutes, stirring at 1-minute intervals.

Variation

For a change of pace, Stephanie suggests replacing the carrots with snow peas, broccoli, cauliflower or green or red bell peppers. Or, to really save time, try using 3 cups (750 mL) frozen Oriental mixed vegetables as a substitute for the onions, carrots, celery and bamboo shoots, reducing stock in Step 1 by 1/4 cup (50 mL).

Sauce

1 1/2 cups	chicken stock	375 mL
1/4 cup	sodium-reduced soya sauce	50 mL
1 tbsp	cornstarch	15 mL
1 tsp	minced garlic	5 mL
1 tsp	granulated sugar	5 mL

Stir-Fry

1 tsp	vegetable oil	5 mL
12 oz	boneless skinless chicken breast, cubed	375g
1 cup	sliced onions	250 mL
1 cup	thinly sliced carrots	250 mL
1/2 cup	chopped celery	125 mL
1	can (6 oz [175 g]) bamboo shoots, drained (optional)	1
1/2 cup	toasted sliced almonds (see Tip at left)	125 mL
8 oz	thin egg noodles	250 g

1. Sauce: In a medium bowl, combine 1 cup (250 mL) of the stock, soya sauce, cornstarch, garlic and sugar. Set aside.

2. In a large nonstick skillet, heat oil over medium-high heat. Add chicken and stir-fry for 6 to 8 minutes or until cooked through. Set aside.

3. Add onions to skillet along with carrots, celery and remaining chicken stock; cook for 4 to 5 minutes. Add bamboo shoots, if using. Add sauce, cooked chicken and almonds; bring to a boil. Reduce heat and simmer for 2 minutes or until thickened.

4. Meanwhile, in a large pot of boiling water, cook noodles until tender but firm; drain. Serve chicken mixture over noodles.

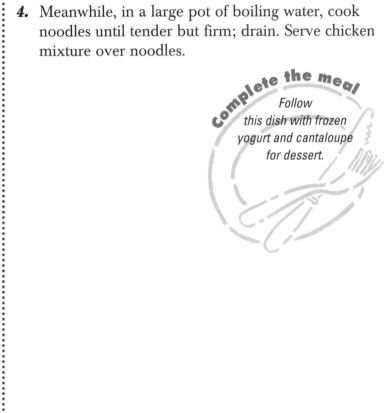

Complete the meal

*Follow
this dish with frozen
yogurt and cantaloupe
for dessert.*

food guide servings

GRAIN PRODUCTS	VEGETABLES & FRUIT
2	1
	1
MILK PRODUCTS	MEAT & ALTERNATIVES

nutrient analysis

PER SERVING			
Calories	465	Carbohydrate	54.7 g
Protein	33.5 g	Dietary Fiber	6.1 g
Fat	12.5 g	Sodium	985 mg

Excellent source of zinc, vitamin A, niacin, vitamin B$_6$. **Good** source of iron, riboflavin, folacin, vitamin B$_{12}$. **Very high** in dietary fiber.

SERVES 4

Lisa Wik
SPRUCE GROVE, AB   P

Creamy Bow-Ties with Chicken, Spinach and Peppers

This attractive dish is perfect for entertaining, but it's so quick and easy you'll want to make it for the family. Kids love it!

TIP

The old Cheddar adds a wonderfully rich flavor to this dish. Other strong-tasting white cheeses, such as Asiago, also work well.

6 oz	bow-tie pasta	175 g
12 oz	boneless skinless chicken breasts, cut into strips	375 g
1 tbsp	vegetable oil	15 mL
1 cup	julienned red bell peppers	250 mL
2 cups	shredded fresh spinach	500 mL
2 tsp	lemon juice	10 mL
1 tbsp	flour	15 mL
1 tsp	minced garlic	5 mL
2 cups	milk	500 mL
1/4 tsp	salt	1 mL
1/4 tsp	nutmeg	1 mL
1/4 tsp	black pepper	1 mL
3/4 cup	shredded old white Cheddar cheese	175 mL
1/4 cup	grated Parmesan cheese	50 mL

1. In a large pot of boiling water, cook pasta until tender but firm; drain. Rinse under hot water; drain. Transfer to a bowl and set aside.

2. Meanwhile, spray a large skillet with vegetable spray. Add chicken strips and cook over medium-high heat for 4 to 5 minutes or until browned and juices run clear when chicken is pierced with a fork. Transfer to a plate.

3. In the same skillet, heat 1 tsp (5 mL) of the oil over medium heat. Add peppers and sauté for 3 to 4 minutes or until slightly softened. Stir in spinach and cook for 1 to 2 minutes or until wilted. Stir in lemon juice. Transfer vegetables to a bowl and set aside.

4. In the same pot used for cooking pasta, heat remaining oil over medium heat; blend in flour. Add garlic and milk; cook, whisking constantly, until mixture comes to a boil. Reduce heat and simmer for 2 to 3 minutes. Stir in salt, nutmeg and pepper. Remove from heat. Add Cheddar cheese and stir until blended. Add pasta, chicken and vegetables to sauce; stir until combined. Serve sprinkled with Parmesan cheese.

Complete the meal

With all four food groups well represented, this dish is the definitive complete meal.

GRAIN PRODUCTS	VEGETABLES & FRUIT
1 1/2	1
1	1
MILK PRODUCTS	MEAT & ALTERNATIVES

nutrient analysis

PER SERVING			
Calories	478	Carbohydrate	42.7 g
Protein	37.9 g	Dietary Fiber	3.0 g
Fat	16.8 g	Sodium	517 mg

Excellent source of vitamin A, vitamin C, thiamin, riboflavin, niacin, vitamin B$_6$, folacin, vitamin B$_{12}$, calcium, iron, zinc. **Moderate** source of dietary fiber.

SERVES 8 — Creole Crockpot Chicken

Enid Witt-Jaques
SASKATOON, SK

Children love the soft chicken and sausage in this recipe – they'll be sure to ask for more.

TIP

If there's someone in your family who, like Enid's husband Doug, prefers a less pronounced tomato flavor in this dish, do what Enid does: substitute 1 can (10 oz [284 mL]) condensed tomato soup for the tomato paste.

2 lbs	skinless boneless chicken thighs	1 kg
2 cups	diced green bell peppers	500 mL
1/2 cup	chopped green onions or cooking onions	125 mL
1	can (19 oz [540 mL]) stewed tomatoes	1
1	can (5.5 oz [155 g]) tomato paste	1
2 tsp	minced garlic	10 mL
1 tsp	hot pepper sauce	5 mL
1	bay leaf	1
2 tsp	dried thyme leaves	10 mL
8 oz	spicy smoked Polish sausage, sliced	250 g

1. Place chicken thighs in bottom of crockpot. Add peppers, onions, tomatoes, tomato paste, garlic, hot pepper sauce, bay leaf and dried thyme. Cook, covered, on Low for 4 to 5 hours. Increase heat setting to High; add sausage and cook for 20 to 30 minutes. Remove bay leaf.

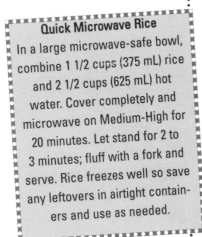

Quick Microwave Rice

In a large microwave-safe bowl, combine 1 1/2 cups (375 mL) rice and 2 1/2 cups (625 mL) hot water. Cover completely and microwave on Medium-High for 20 minutes. Let stand for 2 to 3 minutes; fluff with a fork and serve. Rice freezes well so save any leftovers in airtight containers and use as needed.

complete the meal

Serve with Quick Microwave Rice (see recipe, at left). Have pudding and cookies for dessert.

food guide servings

GRAIN PRODUCTS	VEGETABLES & FRUIT
	2
	1
MILK PRODUCTS	MEAT & ALTERNATIVES

nutrient analysis

PER SERVING			
Calories	284	Carbohydrate	11.7 g
Protein	27.5 g	Dietary Fiber	2.3 g
Fat	14.3 g	Sodium	549 mg

Excellent source of zinc, vitamin C, niacin, vitamin B_6, vitamin B_{12}. **Good** source of iron, thiamin, riboflavin. **Moderate** source of dietary fiber.

EXOTIC GINGER-CUMIN CHICKEN (PAGE 136) ➤
OVERLEAF: QUICK STEAMED FISH FILLETS WITH POTATOES AND ASPARAGUS (PAGE 140)

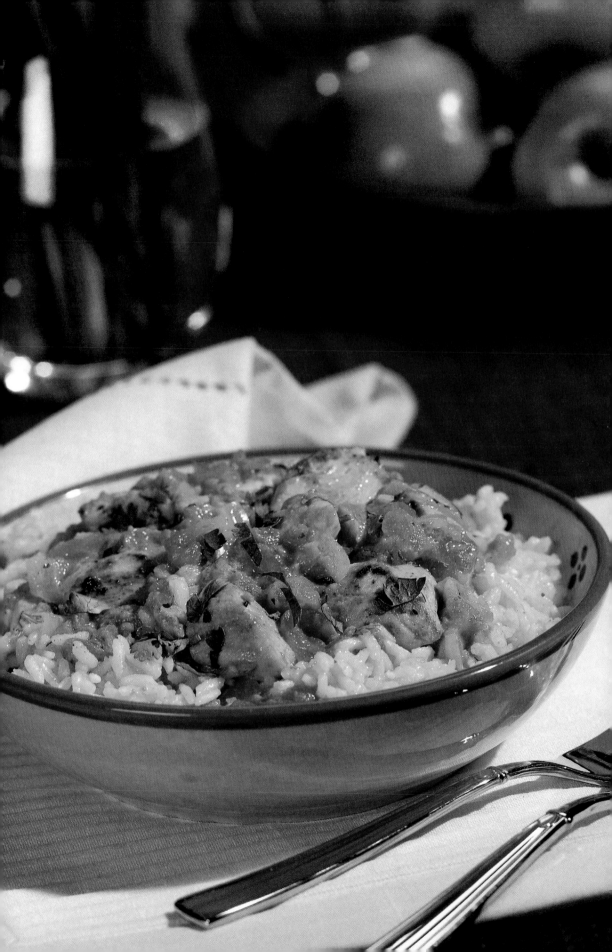

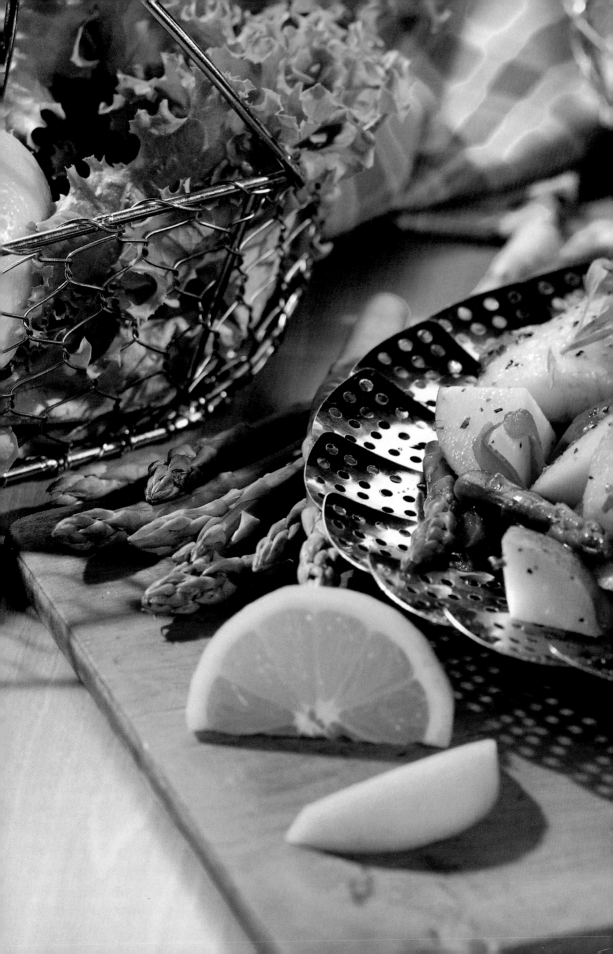

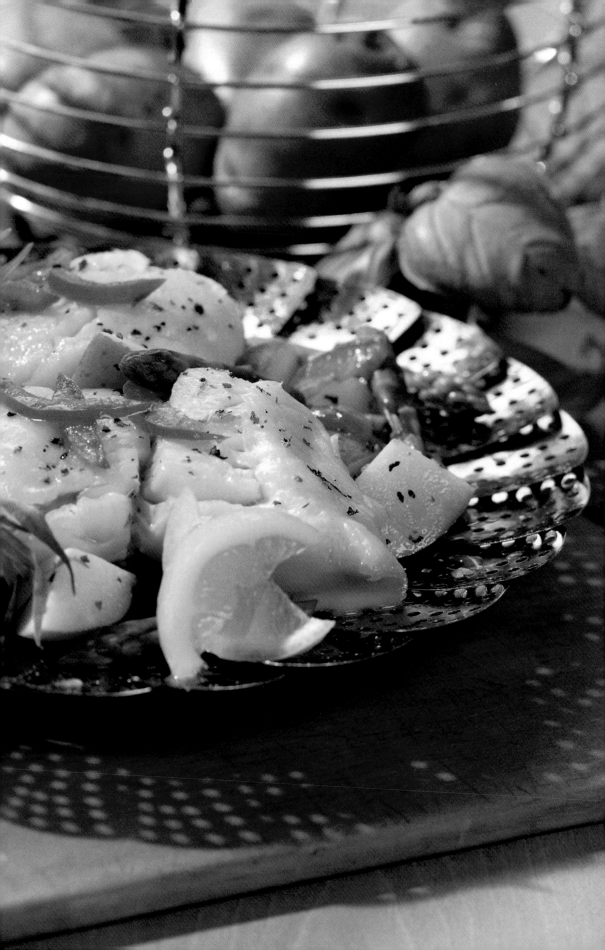

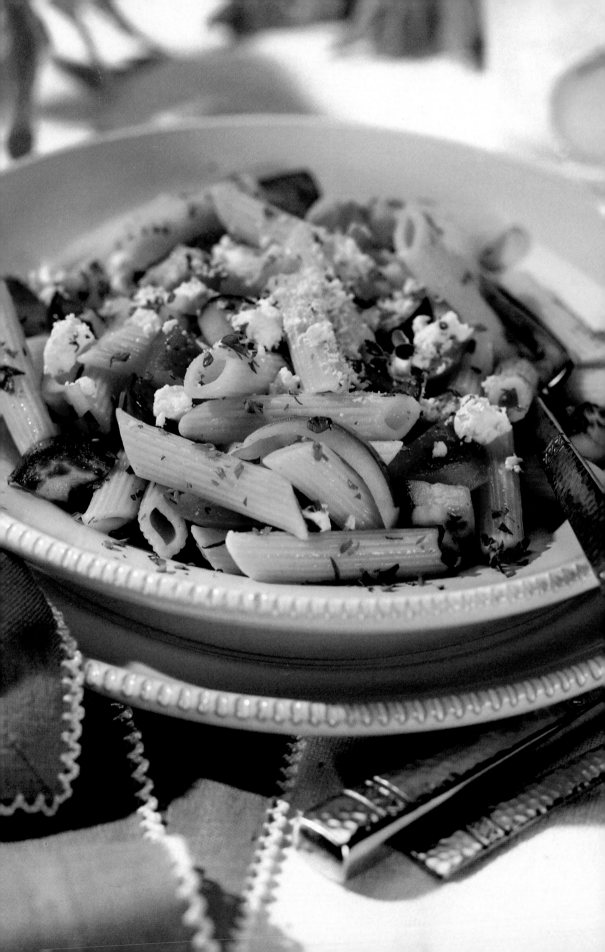

SERVES 6

Ronald Smedmor
NEPEAN, ON [P]

Curried Chicken with Apples and Bananas

Here's a dish from the Kashmir region, where Ronald served for a year in the armed forces. He developed this recipe based on what he learned from the local people.

TIP
Mixing flour with the yogurt prevents it from curdling when added to the hot liquid in the last step of this recipe.

Complete the meal

Serve over brown rice.

2 tbsp	vegetable oil	25 mL
1	3-lb (1.5 kg) chicken, skin removed and cut into 6 to 8 pieces	1
1 cup	chopped onions	250 mL
1 tbsp	minced garlic	15 mL
2 tbsp	mild or medium curry powder	25 mL
2 tsp	ground turmeric	10 mL
1/2 tsp	ground cumin	2 mL
1/2 tsp	ground coriander	2 mL
1 cup	diced peeled tart apples	250 mL
1 1/2 cups	diced bananas	375 mL
1 1/2 cups	diced tomatoes	375 mL
1 cup	chicken stock	250 mL
1 cup	lower-fat plain yogurt	250 mL
	Salt	

1. In a large saucepan or Dutch oven, heat 1 tbsp (15 mL) of the oil over medium-high heat. Add half of the chicken pieces and cook, turning once, until brown. Repeat with remaining oil and chicken. Transfer chicken to a plate and set aside.

2. Reduce heat to medium. Add onions and garlic; cook for 5 minutes or until soft. Stir in curry powder, turmeric, cumin and coriander; sauté for 1 minute.

3. Add apples, bananas, tomatoes and chicken stock; bring to a boil. Reduce heat and simmer, uncovered and stirring frequently, for 5 minutes or until liquid is reduced by half. Return chicken to pan; simmer, covered, for 30 minutes or until juices run clear when chicken is pierced with a fork.

4. Stir in yogurt; simmer for 15 minutes, stirring occasionally. Watch for curdling. Season to taste with salt.

food guide servings

GRAIN PRODUCTS	VEGETABLES & FRUIT
	1
1/4	1
MILK PRODUCTS	MEAT & ALTERNATIVES

nutrient analysis

PER SERVING			
Calories	273	Carbohydrate	19.8 g
Protein	27.7 g	Dietary Fiber	2.2 g
Fat	9.5 g	Sodium	247 mg

Excellent source of zinc, niacin, vitamin B$_6$. **Good** source of riboflavin, vitamin B$_{12}$. **Moderate** source of dietary fiber.

◄ PASTA WITH ROASTED VEGETABLES AND GOAT CHEESE (PAGE 149)

SERVES 6

Curried Red Pepper Chicken

Susanna Law, RD
CALGARY, AB   P

"This meal is a family favorite," Susanna says. *"It's a quick, colorful meal to make when you suddenly find yourself having company for dinner!"*

TIP

This dish is very spicy – so feel free to adjust the curry paste to suit your "fire" tolerance!

2 tsp	vegetable oil	10 mL
1 1/4 lbs	boneless skinless chicken breasts, cut into strips	625 g
1 cup	thinly sliced carrots	250 mL
2 cups	julienned red bell peppers	500 mL
3 tbsp	curry paste	45 mL
1 cup	chicken stock	250 mL
1 tsp	minced garlic	5 mL
1/4 tsp	black pepper	1 mL
1/4 cup	water	50 mL
1 tbsp	cornstarch	15 mL

1. In a large nonstick skillet, heat 1 tsp (5 mL) of the oil over medium-high heat. Add chicken strips and cook for 4 to 5 minutes or until browned on all sides. Remove chicken and set aside.

2. In same skillet, heat remaining oil over medium-high heat. Add carrots and peppers; cook for 3 minutes. Add curry paste and cook, stirring, for 1 minute or until thoroughly combined.

3. Return chicken to skillet. Stir in stock, garlic and pepper; bring to a boil. Reduce heat and simmer for 5 to 6 minutes or until chicken is cooked through and vegetables are tender-crisp.

4. In a small bowl, whisk together water and cornstarch; add to skillet. Cook over medium heat for 1 to 2 minutes or until thickened.

Complete the meal

Susanna suggests serving this delicious curry over Coconut Rice: Just prepare rice using low-fat coconut milk in place of water. Have CUCUMBER RAITA SALAD (see recipe, page 85) on the side.

food guide servings

GRAIN PRODUCTS	VEGETABLES & FRUIT
	1
	1
MILK PRODUCTS	MEAT & ALTERNATIVES

nutrient analysis

PER SERVING			
Calories	183	Carbohydrate	6.9 g
Protein	23.1 g	Dietary Fiber	1.2 g
Fat	6.7 g	Sodium	193 mg

Excellent source of vitamin A, vitamin C, niacin, vitamin B$_6$.
Good source of vitamin B$_{12}$.

SERVES 4

Hot 'n' Spicy Turkey Burgers

Joanne Saunders
SURREY, BC

PREHEAT BARBECUE OR BROILER

These make a nice alternative to the usual beef burgers.

TIP

After brushing uncooked meat with sauce, be sure you don't allow the brush to contact the cooked meat; otherwise, it will become contaminated with harmful bacteria.

Make Ahead
When you have time, double or triple this recipe and freeze the extra patties, uncooked, for up to 3 months.

Complete the meal
Serve with lettuce, tomato and the usual burger fixings. Try SWEET POTATO "FRIES" (see recipe, page 97) or QUICK MARINATED BEAN SALAD (see recipe, page 81) on the side. Finish with ice cream cones.

Sauce

1/2 cup	ketchup	125 mL
1 tbsp	vinegar	15 mL
1 tbsp	Worcestershire sauce	15 mL
2	cloves garlic, minced	2
1/4 to 1/2 tsp	crushed red pepper flakes	1 to 2 mL
1/4 tsp	hot pepper sauce	1 mL
1/4 tsp	black pepper	1 mL

Burgers

1 lb	ground turkey	500 g
1/3 cup	quick-cooking oats	75 mL
4	large hamburger buns, sliced	4

1. **Sauce:** In a small bowl, combine ketchup, vinegar, Worcestershire sauce, garlic, red pepper flakes, hot pepper sauce and pepper. Set aside.

2. **Burgers:** In a large bowl, combine turkey and oats. Add half the sauce; mix thoroughly. Form into 4 large patties.

3. Barbecue on greased grill or broil 6 inches (15 cm) from heat for 5 to 7 minutes per side. Brush with remaining sauce after burgers have been turned.

GRAIN PRODUCTS	VEGETABLES & FRUIT
2 1/2	
MILK PRODUCTS	MEAT & ALTERNATIVES
	1

nutrient analysis

PER SERVING			
Calories	416	Carbohydrate	46.7 g
Protein	26.8 g	Dietary Fiber	2.6 g
Fat	13.5 g	Sodium	832 mg

Excellent source of niacin, folacin, iron, zinc. **Good** source of thiamin, riboflavin, vitamin B_6. **Moderate** source of dietary fiber.

SERVES 6

Skillet Chicken and Shrimp Paella

Kelly Husband
VANCOUVER, BC P

Don't be daunted by the long ingredient list. This one-pot meal is a snap to prepare – the perfect dish for casual entertaining. Kelly has little time as she is a nutrition student at UBC.

Variation

Shrimp can be replaced with 8 oz (250 g) cooked Italian sausage (hot or mild), cut into slices; add to recipe in Step 3 when chicken is returned to skillet. Keep in mind, though, that using sausage will increase the fat content. For an all-chicken dish, substitute an equal amount of additional chicken for the shrimp. Or try a combination of chicken, shrimp and sausage.

1 tbsp	olive oil	15 mL
12 oz	boneless skinless chicken breasts, cut into strips	375 g
1/2 cup	chopped onions	125 mL
2 tsp	minced garlic	10 mL
1	can (10 oz [284 mL]) chicken broth	1
1 1/4 cups	water	300 mL
1	can (19 oz [540 mL]) stewed tomatoes, with juice	1
1 1/4 cups	uncooked long grain rice	300 mL
1 tsp	dried oregano	5 mL
1/2 tsp	paprika	2 mL
1/4 tsp	salt	1 mL
1/4 tsp	black pepper	1 mL
1/4 tsp	ground turmeric *or* crumbled saffron	1 mL
1 cup	julienned red bell peppers	250 mL
1 cup	snow peas, trimmed and cut into bite-size pieces *or* frozen peas	250 mL
8 oz	cooked large shrimp (about 15)	250 g

1. In a large nonstick skillet, heat 2 tsp (10 mL) of the oil over medium-high heat. Add chicken and cook until browned and no longer pink inside. Remove from pan and set aside.

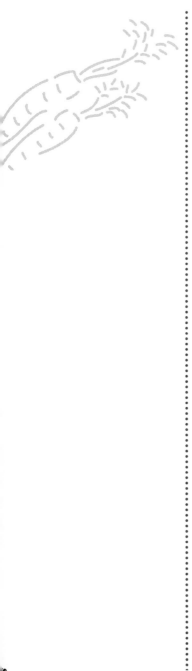

2. In the same skillet, heat remaining oil over medium-high heat. Add onions; reduce heat to medium and cook for 3 to 4 minutes or until softened but not brown. Add garlic, broth, water, tomatoes, rice, oregano, paprika, salt, pepper and turmeric; bring to a boil. Reduce heat and simmer, covered, for 15 minutes.

3. Add red peppers and simmer, covered, for 4 to 5 minutes or until rice is tender. Stir in snow peas, cooked chicken and shrimp; simmer, uncovered, for 2 to 3 minutes or until heated through.

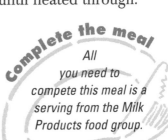

complete the meal

All you need to compete this meal is a serving from the Milk Products food group.

food guide servings

GRAIN PRODUCTS	VEGETABLES & FRUIT
1 1/2	1 1/2
	1
MILK PRODUCTS	MEAT & ALTERNATIVES

nutrient analysis

PER SERVING			
Calories	317	Carbohydrate	40.4 g
Protein	27.6 g	Dietary Fiber	2.3 g
Fat	4.6 g	Sodium	775 mg

Excellent source of vitamin C, niacin, vitamin B$_6$, vitamin B$_{12}$. **Good** source of iron, zinc, vitamin A. **Moderate** source of dietary fiber.

SERVES 6

Adapted from
The Dairy Farmers of Canada P

Turkey Pot Pie with Biscuit Topping

PREHEAT OVEN TO 400° F (200° C)
12-CUP (3 L) DEEP BAKING DISH, GREASED

There's nothing better than a pot pie when you need to use up leftover turkey or chicken. If you don't have leftovers, purchase a cooked chicken at your grocery store or roast your own turkey breast. Roast one large bone-in turkey breast (2 lbs [1 kg]) at 350° F (180° C) for 70 to 80 minutes or until juices run clear and thermometer registers 170° F (77° C); immediately transfer to the refrigerator and keep for up to 3 days.

3 tbsp	butter	45 mL
2 cups	sliced mushrooms	500 mL
1/4 cup	flour	50 mL
1 cup	chicken stock	250 mL
2 cups	milk	500 mL
2 tbsp	sherry (optional)	25 mL
1/2 tsp	ground thyme	2 mL
1/2 tsp	ground sage	2 mL
1/2 tsp	salt	2 mL
3 cups	cubed cooked turkey breast	750 mL
4 cups	frozen mixed vegetables	1 L
	Freshly ground black pepper	

Biscuit Topping

1 1/2 cups	biscuit baking mix	375 mL
1 tsp	dried parsley	5 mL
7 tbsp	milk	105 mL

1. In a large saucepan, melt 1 tbsp (15 mL) of the butter over medium heat. Add mushrooms and cook for 4 to 5 minutes or until moisture has evaporated, but do not brown. Add remaining butter to pan; stir in flour and blend well. Whisk in stock, milk and, if using, sherry. Stir in thyme, sage and salt; bring to a boil. Reduce heat to low and cook, stirring constantly, for 3 to 5 minutes or until thickened. Remove from heat.

2. Stir in turkey and frozen vegetables. Season to taste with pepper. Spoon into prepared baking dish.

3. Biscuit Topping: In a bowl combine biscuit mix with parsley; stir in 6 tbsp (75 mL) milk. Gather dough into a ball, adding more baking mix as required to make dough easy to handle. On a lightly floured surface roll out dough to fit top of baking dish; place over filling. Cut a small vent hole in center of topping. Brush with remaining 1 tbsp (15 mL) milk.

4. Bake in preheated oven for 35 to 40 minutes or until topping is golden and casserole is bubbling hot.

Complete the meal

This fabulous four-food-group dish is a complete meal on its own.

food guide servings

GRAIN PRODUCTS	VEGETABLES & FRUIT
1 1/2	1 1/2
1/4	1
MILK PRODUCTS	MEAT & ALTERNATIVES

nutrient analysis

PER SERVING			
Calories	434	Carbohydrate	45.1 g
Protein	31.5 g	Dietary Fiber	5.3 g
Fat	14.2 g	Sodium	808 mg

Excellent source of iron, zinc, vitamin A, riboflavin, niacin, vitamin B_6. **Good** source of calcium, thiamin, folacin, vitamin B_{12}. **High** in dietary fiber.

SERVES 8

Marcella Maclellan
NEW GLASGOW, NS [P]

Exotic Ginger-Cumin Chicken

TIP

Canola oil is high in monounsaturated fat and very low in saturated fat. It is inexpensive and widely available. And because of its neutral flavor, it is an excellent all-purpose oil for baking, cooking and salad dressings.

Complete the meal

Serve over basmati rice with a cool, creamy CUCUMBER RAITA SALAD (see recipe, page 85) and pappadums or naan.

Quick Microwave Broccoli

Place 1 lb (500 g) broccoli, stems facing outwards, in a round microwave-safe dish; sprinkle with 1 tbsp (15 mL) water. Cover with vented plastic wrap and microwave on High for 5 to 6 minutes. Let stand for 2 minutes.

1 tbsp	vegetable oil	15 mL
2 lbs	boneless skinless chicken breasts, cut into bite-size pieces	1 kg
2 tsp	minced garlic	10 mL
1/2 cup	chopped onion	125 mL
1 tbsp	finely chopped ginger root or 1/2 tsp (2 mL) ground ginger	15 mL
1/4 to 1/2 tsp	cayenne pepper	1 to 2 mL
1 tsp	ground coriander	5 mL
1 tsp	ground cumin	5 mL
1 tsp	ground turmeric	5 mL
1/2 cup	chicken stock	125 mL
1	can (19 oz [540 mL]) stewed tomatoes	1
2 tbsp	tomato paste	25 mL
2 tsp	granulated sugar	10 mL
1/2 tsp	salt	2 mL
3/4 cup	lower-fat plain yogurt	175 mL
2 tbsp	chopped fresh coriander (optional)	25 mL

1. In large saucepan or Dutch oven, heat 2 tsp (10 mL) of the oil over medium high heat. Add half the chicken and cook for 2 to 3 minutes or until brown. Remove from pan and set aside. Repeat with remaining chicken.

2. Add remaining oil to pan; add garlic, onion and ginger. Reduce heat to medium and cook, stirring constantly, for 4 to 5 minutes until softened, but not brown. Stir in cayenne, coriander, cumin and turmeric. Sauté for 1 minute or until fragrant.

3. Stir in stock, tomatoes, tomato paste, sugar and salt; return chicken to pan. Bring to a boil; reduce heat and simmer for 5 minutes until chicken is cooked through.

4. Stir in yogurt and coriander and simmer over very low heat for 1 to 2 minutes.

food guide servings

GRAIN PRODUCTS	VEGETABLES & FRUIT
	1
	1
MILK PRODUCTS	MEAT & ALTERNATIVES

nutrient analysis

PER SERVING			
Calories	193	Carbohydrate	9.9 g
Protein	28.4 g	Dietary Fiber	1.2 g
Fat	4.2 g	Sodium	454 mg

Excellent source of niacin, vitamin B6. **Good** source of vitamin B12.

Diana Stenlund-Moffat, RD
BRUCE MINES, ON

SERVES 4

Crunchy Fish Burgers

PREHEAT OVEN TO 375° F (190° C)
BAKING SHEET, GREASED

These are fairly substantial burgers, so serve them with something light. For young children, half a burger will probably be enough.

Nutrition Facts

The deep-fried fish sandwiches or burgers typically served at fast food restaurants are loaded with fat – some have more than twice that of a cheeseburger! With these fish burgers, however, the fat content is about the same as that of a plain hamburger.

Variation

"Crunchy Fried Chicken" Burgers: Substitute 3 lbs (1.5 kg) skinless bone-in chicken thighs and legs for the fish. Prepare coating as for fish fillets, but bake in preheated oven for 30 to 35 minutes or until juices run clear when pierced with a fork.

Complete the meal

Serve with raw vegetables and Herbed Yogurt Dip (see recipe, page 50).

Crunchy Coating

1 cup	crushed corn flakes	250 mL
1/2 tsp	garlic powder	2 mL
1/2 tsp	dry mustard	2 mL
1/4 tsp	black pepper	1 mL

Burgers

1	egg	1
1 tbsp	water	15 mL
1 lb	fresh or frozen fish fillets (sole, perch or halibut), patted dry	500 g

Zippy Tartar Sauce

1/4 cup	sweet pickle or dill pickle relish	50 mL
2 tbsp	light mayonnaise	25 mL
1/4 tsp	horseradish	1 mL
4	6-inch (15 cm) submarine-type buns, sliced	4
4	lettuce leaves	4
2	medium tomatoes, sliced	2

1. Crunchy Coating: In a heavy plastic bag, combine crumbs, garlic powder, mustard and pepper.

2. Burgers: In a shallow bowl, lightly beat together egg and water; set aside. Dip fish fillets in egg mixture and transfer, one piece at a time, to plastic bag; shake gently to coat. Place on baking sheet. Bake in preheated oven for 10 to 15 minutes or until fish is opaque and flakes easily with a fork.

3. Zippy Tartar Sauce: In a small bowl, blend together relish, mayonnaise and horseradish.

4. Assembly: Spread buns with tartar sauce; add fish fillets and top with lettuce and tomato.

food guide servings

GRAIN PRODUCTS	VEGETABLES & FRUIT
3 1/2	1/2
	1
MILK PRODUCTS	MEAT & ALTERNATIVES

nutrient analysis

PER SERVING			
Calories	503	Carbohydrate	71.7 g
Protein	31.9 g	Dietary Fiber	3.4 g
Fat	9.5 g	Sodium	894 mg

Excellent source of thiamin, niacin, vitamin B$_6$, folacin, vitamin B$_{12}$, iron. **Good** source of riboflavin, zinc. **Moderate** source of dietary fiber.

SERVES 4

Marilena Rutka
TORONTO, ON Ⓟ

Parmesan-Herb Baked Fish Fillets

This elegant entrée is one that Marilena often serves when entertaining. For convenience and speed, we use frozen fish fillets here. But Marilena uses a thicker fish fillet such as salmon or halibut and increases the cooking time by about 5 minutes.

TIP

Substitute 1 to 2 tbsp (15 to 25 mL) chopped fresh basil for the dried basil.

It is important to use dried bread crumbs; fresh bread crumbs will make the dish too soggy.

Nutrition Facts

Fish fillets that are light in color – such as haddock, halibut, sole and cod – tend to be lower in fat than darker-colored fillets from fish such as salmon, mackerel, tuna, herring and rainbow trout.

PREHEAT OVEN TO 400° F (200° C)
11- BY 7-INCH (2 L) BAKING DISH, GREASED

1	package (1 lb [500 g]) frozen fish fillets, thawed and patted dry	1
1/4 cup	light mayonnaise	50 mL
1/4 cup	grated Parmesan cheese	50 mL
2 tbsp	chopped green onions	25 mL
1 tbsp	chopped pimento or red bell pepper	15 mL
	Cayenne pepper to taste	
1/2 cup	dried bread crumbs	125 mL
1/2 tsp	dried basil	2 mL
	Black pepper to taste	

1. Place fish fillets in a single layer in bottom of prepared baking dish. Set aside.

2. In a small bowl, stir together mayonnaise, Parmesan cheese, onions, pimento and cayenne pepper. Spread mixture evenly over fish fillets.

3. In a separate bowl, combine bread crumbs, basil and pepper; sprinkle over top of fish. Bake in preheated oven for 10 to 12 minutes or until fish is opaque and flakes easily with a fork.

Complete the meal

Serve with SAUTÉED SPINACH WITH PINE NUTS (see recipe, page 99) and boiled new potatoes. Have PEACH COBBLER (see recipe, page 169) for dessert.

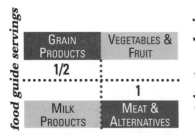

food guide servings

GRAIN PRODUCTS	VEGETABLES & FRUIT
1/2	
	1
MILK PRODUCTS	MEAT & ALTERNATIVES

nutrient analysis

PER SERVING			
Calories	216	Carbohydrate	11.9 g
Protein	23.3 g	Dietary Fiber	0.3 g
Fat	7.8 g	Sodium	383 mg

Excellent source of niacin, vitamin B$_{12}$.
Good source of vitamin B$_6$.

Mary Anne Pucovsky
AILSA CRAIG, ON

Pasta with White Clam Sauce

"This pasta dish is very fast and delicious," Mary Anne says. She suggests preparing the sauce first and then cooking the pasta just before serving, since the cappellini cooks very quickly.

TIP

Fresh clams are superb in this dish. Substitute 2 cups (500 mL) fresh shucked clams for the canned clams. Instead of the reserved clam juice, use 3/4 cup (175 mL) fish or vegetable stock.

Nutrition Facts

For recipes that call for cream, try replacing it with evaporated milk – it's lower in fat and contains more calcium. Keep some handy in your pantry.

Variation

For a change of color, try making this pasta with red clam sauce: Just add 1 cup (250 mL) chopped tomatoes to the sauce at the end of Step 1.

1 tbsp	olive oil	15 mL
1/4 cup	chopped onions	50 mL
2 cups	sliced mushrooms	500 mL
2 tsp	flour	10 mL
1/3 cup	dry white wine	75 mL
2	cans (each 5 oz [142 g]) clams, drained, reserving 3/4 cup (175 mL) clam juice	2
1 tsp	minced garlic	5 mL
1	can (5 1/2 oz [160 mL]) evaporated 2% milk	1
1/8 tsp	ground nutmeg	0.5 mL
8 oz	cappellini *or* vermicelli	250 g
2 tbsp	freshly chopped parsley (or 2 tsp [10 mL] dried)	25 mL
	Black pepper	

1. In a large nonstick skillet, heat oil over medium-high heat. Add onions and mushrooms; sauté for 5 to 6 minutes or until softened and moisture has evaporated. Sprinkle with flour; blend well. Add wine, reserved clam juice and garlic; bring to a boil. Reduce heat and simmer for 2 to 3 minutes or until thickened. Stir in clams, evaporated milk and nutmeg; simmer for 1 to 2 minutes or until heated through.

2. Just before serving, cook pasta according to package directions or until tender but firm; drain. Toss with sauce. Sprinkle with parsley. Season to taste with pepper.

Complete the meal
Serve with any green salad and your favorite vinaigrette dressing.

GRAIN PRODUCTS	VEGETABLES & FRUIT
2	1/2
1/4	1
MILK PRODUCTS	MEAT & ALTERNATIVES

nutrient analysis

PER SERVING			
Calories	412	Carbohydrate	54.4 g
Protein	29.5 g	Dietary Fiber	3.2 g
Fat	6.8 g	Sodium	227 mg

Excellent source of iron, zinc, thiamin, riboflavin, niacin, folacin. **Good** source of calcium, vitamin A, vitamin C. **Moderate** source of dietary fiber.

SERVES 2

Quick Steamed Fish Fillets with Potatoes and Asparagus

N. Schneider
WINNIPEG, MB

This elegant supper for two is simplicity itself. The entire meal is prepared in a steamer and ready in 15 minutes.

TIP
Substitute 1 to 2 tsp (5 to 10 mL) of your favorite fresh herbs for the dried herbs.

If asparagus is out of season, use fresh green beans instead.

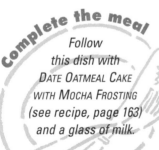

Nutrition Facts
Steaming is a fast, efficient and low-fat way to prepare fish. It's also a great way to cook vegetables so that they're crisp and retain their nutrients.

Complete the meal
Follow this dish with DATE OATMEAL CAKE WITH MOCHA FROSTING *(see recipe, page 163) and a glass of milk.*

1 cup	small new red potatoes, quartered	250 mL
1 cup	asparagus, cut into 1-inch (2.5 cm) pieces	250 mL
2	4-oz (125 g) fish fillets, about 1 inch (2.5 cm) thick	2
1/3 cup	julienned tomatoes (preferably Roma)	75 mL
1/4 to 1/2 tsp	dried basil or tarragon	1 to 2 mL
	Black pepper to taste	
1 tsp	butter	5 mL
1 tsp	lemon juice	5 mL
	Salt	

1. Place potatoes in a large steamer set over a pot of boiling water. Cover and steam for 8 to 10 minutes or until potatoes are beginning to soften but are not yet cooked.

2. Place asparagus on top of potatoes. Place fish fillets on top of asparagus. Top with tomatoes; sprinkle with basil and pepper. Cover and steam for 5 to 6 minutes or until fish is opaque and flakes easily with a fork. Dot with butter; cover and steam for 30 seconds or until butter is melted. Sprinkle with lemon juice. Season to taste with salt.

food guide servings

GRAIN PRODUCTS	VEGETABLES & FRUIT
	2
	1
MILK PRODUCTS	MEAT & ALTERNATIVES

nutrient analysis

PER SERVING			
Calories	183	Carbohydrate	14.5 g
Protein	24.8 g	Dietary Fiber	2.5 g
Fat	3.0 g	Sodium	110 mg

Excellent source of niacin, vitamin B$_6$, folacin, vitamin B$_{12}$. **Good** source of iron, vitamin C. **Moderate** source of dietary fiber.

SERVES 2

Lynn Roblin, RD

Salmon with Roasted Vegetables

PREHEAT OVEN TO 425° F (220° C)
11- BY 7-INCH (2 L) BAKING DISH

1 tbsp	olive oil	15 mL
2 tsp	minced garlic	10 mL
2 tsp	dried thyme	10 mL
1 cup	diced peeled sweet potatoes	250 mL
1 cup	diced zucchini or red bell peppers	250 mL
1 cup	diced peeled parsnips or potatoes	250 mL
2 tbsp	lemon juice	25 mL
1/4 tsp	black pepper	1 mL
1	salmon tail (8 to 12 oz [250 to 375 g]), patted dry	1

TIP

Here's a great dish for parents who want to savor a quiet meal together after the children have been fed and put to bed. With or without the kids, it's a perfect meal for two.

We use the tail end of the salmon here, since it contains the fewest bones. However, you can substitute two 4-oz (125 g) salmon fillets.

Nutrition Facts
This salmon dish is relatively high in fat. To balance your meal, serve with lower-fat accompaniments.

1. In a small bowl, stir together olive oil, garlic and 1 tsp (5 mL) of the thyme. Place sweet potatoes, zucchini and parsnips in baking dish and sprinkle with oil mixture; toss to coat. Spread out vegetables in a single layer and roast in preheated oven for 15 minutes.

2. In the bowl used for oil mixture, combine remaining thyme, lemon juice and pepper. Brush mixture over salmon tail.

3. Remove vegetables from oven and stir. Place salmon, skin-side down, on top of vegetables. Bake for 10 to 15 minutes or until fish is opaque and flakes easily with a fork. Remove skin from salmon before serving.

complete the meal

Serve this meal with brown rice or Quick Couscous (see recipe, page 118). Finish the meal with frozen yogurt.

GRAIN PRODUCTS	VEGETABLES & FRUIT
	3
	1
MILK PRODUCTS	MEAT & ALTERNATIVES

nutrient analysis

PER SERVING			
Calories	415	Carbohydrate	34.4 g
Protein	25.3 g	Dietary Fiber	5.1 g
Fat	20.0 g	Sodium	84 mg

Excellent source of vitamin A, vitamin C, thiamin, niacin, vitamin B$_6$, folacin, vitamin B$_{12}$. **Good** source of riboflavin, iron. **High** in dietary fiber.

SERVES 4 Shrimp and Mussels with Couscous

Johanne Trepanier
BROMONT, PQ

Here's a dish that Johanne tells us is as delicious as it is easy to make! The couscous makes a great accompaniment – and it's ready in minutes.

TIP

Mussels should be rinsed in several changes of cold water to rid them of any grit.

Inspect mussels before cooking and discard any with shells that are broken or do not close: these are not safe to eat. Likewise, discard any mussels that do not open after cooking.

1 tbsp	olive oil	15 mL
1 cup	sliced leeks, green and white parts	250 mL
1/2 cup	diced carrots	125 mL
1	can (19 oz [540 mL]) stewed tomatoes	1
1 tsp	minced garlic	5 mL
1 cup	green bell pepper strips	250 mL
1 lb	fresh mussels, cleaned	500 g
1 1/2 cups	quick-cooking couscous	375 mL
12	large cooked shrimp	12

1. In a large saucepan or Dutch oven, heat oil over medium-high heat. Add leeks and sauté for 2 to 3 minutes. Add carrots, tomatoes and garlic; bring to a boil. Cover, reduce heat and simmer for 10 minutes.

2. Add green pepper strips and mussels; cook, covered, for 5 minutes or until mussels have opened. Discard any mussels that do not open.

3. Meanwhile, cook couscous according to package directions.

4. Add shrimp to mussel mixture; cook for 2 minutes or until heated through. Serve over couscous.

Complete the meal

Finish off your meal with fresh berries and ice cream.

food guide servings

GRAIN PRODUCTS	VEGETABLES & FRUIT
2	2 1/2
	1/2
MILK PRODUCTS	MEAT & ALTERNATIVES

nutrient analysis

PER SERVING			
Calories	390	Carbohydrate	68.8 g
Protein	18 g	Dietary Fiber	5.7 g
Fat	5 g	Sodium	489 mg

Excellent source of iron, vitamin C, vitamin A, niacin, folacin, vitamin B_{12}. **Good** source of zinc, thiamin, vitamin B_6. **High** in dietary fiber.

Spaghettini with Tuna, Olives and Capers

Laurie A. Wadsworth, PDt
ANTIGONISH, NS

SERVES 4

8 to 12 oz	spaghettini	250 to 375 g
2 tsp	olive oil	10 mL
1/2 cup	chopped onions	125 mL
5	anchovies (optional)	5
3 cups	PIQUANT TOMATO SAUCE (see recipe, page 150) *or* commercially prepared pasta sauce	750 mL
1	can (6 oz [170 g]) tuna, drained	1
1/2 cup	sliced black olives	125 mL
2 tbsp	drained capers	25 mL
1/4 cup	chopped fresh basil (or 1 tsp [5 mL] dried)	50 mL

1. In a large pot of boiling water, cook pasta until tender but firm; drain.

2. In a large nonstick skillet, heat oil over medium-high heat. Add onions and sauté for 3 to 4 minutes or until softened. Add anchovies, if using, and cook for 1 to 2 minutes or until dissolved into a paste.

3. Stir in PIQUANT TOMATO SAUCE, tuna, olives and capers; bring to a boil. Reduce heat and simmer for 5 minutes. Stir in basil and cook for 1 minute. Serve over pasta.

complete the meal
This is almost a complete meal – all it needs is a glass of milk.

food guide servings

GRAIN PRODUCTS	VEGETABLES & FRUIT
2	2 1/2
	1/2
MILK PRODUCTS	MEAT & ALTERNATIVES

nutrient analysis

PER SERVING			
Calories	390	Carbohydrate	60.6 g
Protein	19.0 g	Dietary Fiber	6.5 g
Fat	8.8 g	Sodium	491 mg

Excellent source of vitamin C, thiamin, riboflavin, niacin, folacin, vitamin B_6, vitamin B_{12}, iron. **Good** source of vitamin A, zinc. **Very high** in dietary fiber.

SERVES 4 — Tuna and Rice Casserole

Marilyn Townshend
SOURIS, PEI

P

PREHEAT OVEN TO 350° F (180° C)
8-INCH (2 L) BAKING DISH, GREASED

Here's a delicious change from the usual tuna noodle casserole – and it takes less than 10 minutes to prepare! It's easy enough for older children and teens to make on their own; younger children can help by grating the cheese and getting the salad ready.

Food Fast

If you don't have time to make a salad, buy ready-to-eat salad at the supermarket.

Nutrition Facts

To reduce fat, buy tuna packed in water – not vegetable oil.

Instead of regular cream of mushroom soup, try a reduced-fat variety.

1	can (10 oz [284 mL]) cream of mushroom soup	1
1 1/4 cups	instant rice	300 mL
1 cup	milk	250 mL
1/2 cup	water	125 mL
1	can (6 oz [170 g]) tuna packed in water, drained	1
1 cup	frozen peas	250 mL
1/4 cup	finely chopped onions	50 mL
1 tsp	lemon juice	5 mL
	Black pepper to taste	
1/2 cup	grated Cheddar cheese	125 mL
	Paprika to taste	

1. In a large bowl, stir together soup, rice, milk, water, tuna, peas, onions, lemon juice and pepper. Pour into prepared baking dish. Sprinkle with cheese and paprika. Bake in preheated oven for 30 to 35 minutes or until bubbling and rice is tender.

Complete the meal

Serve this casserole with any green salad and your favorite vinaigrette dressing.

food guide servings

GRAIN PRODUCTS	VEGETABLES & FRUIT
1	1/2
1/2	1/2
MILK PRODUCTS	MEAT & ALTERNATIVES

nutrient analysis

PER SERVING			
Calories	330	Carbohydrate	35.1 g
Protein	19.4 g	Dietary Fiber	2.2 g
Fat	12.1 g	Sodium	874 mg

Excellent source of niacin, vitamin B_{12}. **Good** source of calcium, zinc, thiamin, riboflavin, vitamin B_6. **Moderate** source of dietary fiber.

SERVES 6

Shannon Crocker, RD
HAMILTON, ON

Chickpea Hot Pot

This is a quick and easy vegetarian dish that's helpful for anyone who needs to increase their intake of folacin, calcium and iron.

TIP

Toss in whatever vegetables you have handy to make your own hot pot variations. You can substitute black beans or red kidney beans for the chickpeas.

Nutrition Facts

Tofu is a creamy white soy product sold in small blocks. It come in different forms: soft or silken (for shakes, dressing, desserts), firm or semi-firm; choose one that suits your needs. On its own, tofu is very bland. When cooked with other ingredients, however, it absorbs their flavors wonderfully. Use tofu in soups, chili, pasta dishes and dips

Tofu is high in protein and makes a good substitute for meat but it also contains fat. A 3 1/2 oz (100 g) serving of tofu made with calcium sulfate provides 77 calories, 8.0 g protein, 5 g fat and 162 mg calcium.

2 tsp	olive oil	10 mL
1/2 cup	chopped onions	125 mL
1 tbsp	curry paste	15 mL
2	cans (each 28 oz [796 mL]) diced plum tomatoes, with juice	2
1	can (19 oz [540 mL]) chickpeas, rinsed and drained	1
1 cup	diced sweet potatoes	250 mL
1 tbsp	granulated sugar	15 mL
1 tsp	minced garlic	5 mL
1 cup	cubed firm tofu	250 mL
2 cups	bok choy, cut into strips	500 mL
2 cups	broccoli florets	500 mL
1/2 tsp	black pepper	2 mL

1. In a large saucepan or Dutch oven, heat oil over medium-high heat. Add onions and cook until softened. Stir in curry paste. Add canned tomatoes, chickpeas, sweet potatoes, sugar and garlic; bring to a boil. Reduce heat and simmer, covered, for 12 to 15 minutes or until sweet potatoes are tender.

2. Stir in tofu, bok choy, broccoli and pepper. Cook, uncovered, for 2 minutes or until broccoli is tender-crisp. Adjust seasoning to taste (add a bit more curry paste if you like it hot).

Complete the meal

Serve with whole grain bread.

nutrient analysis

GRAIN PRODUCTS	VEGETABLES & FRUIT
	4
	1
MILK PRODUCTS	MEAT & ALTERNATIVES

PER SERVING			
Calories	229	Carbohydrate	37.2 g
Protein	10.9 g	Dietary Fiber	6.5 g
Fat	5.8 g	Sodium	592 mg

Excellent source of vitamin A, vitamin C, folacin and vitamin B$_6$. **Good** source of calcium, iron, zinc, thiamin and niacin. **Very high** in dietary fiber.

SERVES 6 Creamy Pasta and Broccoli

Esther Murphy
SIDNEY, BC

*This may be just the recipe
you need to convert your
children into broccoli-lovers!*

Nutrition Facts

If your children won't eat
vegetables, don't force them
– but don't give up either!
Continue to offer a variety of
vegetables in single, one-bite
servings. Tastes change and
some children simply take
longer to accept certain
foods.

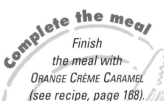

Complete the meal

*Finish
the meal with
ORANGE CRÈME CARAMEL
(see recipe, page 168).*

12 oz	penne or macaroni or other pasta	375 g
3 cups	chopped broccoli (fresh or frozen)	750 mL
1 tbsp	butter *or* margarine	15 mL
1 tbsp	flour	15 mL
1 1/2 cups	chicken stock *or* vegetable stock	375 mL
1 tsp	minced garlic	5 mL
1	package (4 oz [125 g]) light herb-and-garlic-flavored cream cheese	1
	Black pepper	
6 tbsp	Parmesan cheese	90 mL

1. In a large pot of boiling water, cook pasta until tender but still firm, adding broccoli during last 3 minutes of cooking time; drain. Set aside.

2. Meanwhile, in a medium saucepan, melt butter over medium heat. Add flour and stir until blended. Whisk in stock. Add garlic and cook, stirring constantly, for 4 to 5 minutes or until thickened. Remove from heat; stir in cream cheese until melted. Season to taste with pepper.

3. Toss pasta and broccoli with sauce. Top each serving with 1 tbsp (15 mL) Parmesan cheese.

food guide servings

GRAIN PRODUCTS	VEGETABLES & FRUIT
2	1
1/4	
MILK PRODUCTS	MEAT & ALTERNATIVES

nutrient analysis

PER SERVING			
Calories	334	Carbohydrate	47.2 g
Protein	13.9 g	Dietary Fiber	3.5 g
Fat	9.8 g	Sodium	438 mg

Excellent source of vitamin C, thiamin, riboflavin, niacin, folacin. **Good** source of iron and folacin. **Moderate** source of dietary fiber.

SERVES 6

Marilynn Small
Post Cereals
TORONTO, ON

P

Crowd-Pleasing Vegetarian Chili

Nutrition Facts

Many adults and children don't get enough fiber in their diet – but they will after a bowl of this nutrient-packed chili. Remember that when adding more fiber to your meals, you should be sure to drink plenty of water to help the fiber work properly.

Complete the meal

Serve this delicious fiber-rich chili with rice, accompanied by a crisp garden salad and lemon or lime sherbet for dessert.

1 tbsp	vegetable oil	15 mL
1	onion, chopped	1
1	red bell pepper, chopped	1
2	cloves garlic, minced	2
1	stalk celery, chopped	1
1 to 2 tbsp	chili powder	15 to 25 mL
2 tsp	ground cumin	10 mL
1	can (28 oz [796 mL]) tomatoes	1
1	can (14 oz [398 mL]) black or red kidney beans, rinsed and drained	1
1	can (12 oz [355 mL]) corn kernels, drained	1
1 cup	bran cereal	250 mL
3 cups	cooked rice	750 mL
1/2 cup	grated Cheddar cheese	125 mL

1. In a large saucepan, heat oil over medium-high heat. Add onion, red pepper, garlic and celery; cook until vegetables are tender. Stir in chili powder and cumin; cook for 1 minute.

2. Add tomatoes, breaking up with spoon. Stir in beans, corn and cereal; bring to a boil. Reduce heat, cover and simmer for 5 minutes. Serve over rice, sprinkled with cheese.

GRAIN PRODUCTS	VEGETABLES & FRUIT
1 1/2	2
	1/2
MILK PRODUCTS	MEAT & ALTERNATIVES

nutrient analysis

PER SERVING			
Calories	366	Carbohydrate	68.3 g
Protein	13.7 g	Dietary Fiber	10.4 g
Fat	7.1 g	Sodium	638 mg

Excellent source of iron, zinc, vitamin C, thiamin, niacin, vitamin B$_6$ and folacin. **Good** source of vitamin A. **Very high** in dietary fiber.

SERVES 4

Fettuccine Carbonara

*Adapted from
Canadian Egg Marketing Agency*

*In taste tests, this has proved
to be a very popular recipe.
It's easy to make and quick
to eat. It's perfect for those
nights when you have to rush
out again after supper.*

TIP

Always be sure to use fresh,
clean eggs with no cracks.

Nutrition Facts

The next time you're buying
groceries, look for omega-3
enriched eggs. While more
expensive than regular eggs,
they are also lower in saturated fat, higher in omega-3
fatty acids and contain more
vitamin E.

12 oz	fettuccine	350 g
4	eggs	4
1 cup	grated Parmesan cheese	250 mL
1/4 cup	chopped fresh parsley (or 1 tbsp [15 mL] dried)	50 mL
1/2 tsp	butter	2 mL
1/2 cup	finely chopped onions	125 mL
1/4 cup	chopped cooked ham *or* crumbled cooked bacon	50 mL
1/8 tsp	black pepper	0.5 mL

1. In a large pot of boiling water, cook fettuccine
according to package directions or until tender but
firm. Drain, reserving about 1/2 cup (125 mL) pasta
cooking water. Return fettuccine to pot.

2. In a medium bowl, whisk together eggs, 3/4 cup
(175 mL) of the Parmesan cheese and parsley. Set
aside.

3. Meanwhile, in a small nonstick skillet, melt butter
over medium heat. Add onions and cook until soft
and transparent. Stir in ham.

4. Add egg mixture to hot pasta; toss until
eggs thicken and coat fettuccine.
Stir in onions and ham. If sauce
is too thick, add reserved
pasta cooking water, a little
bit at a time, stirring, until
desired consistency is
reached. Serve piping hot,
sprinkled with remaining
Parmesan cheese and pepper.

Complete the meal

*Serve
with a tossed green
salad and a low-fat salad
dressing, or a green
vegetable.*

food guide servings

GRAIN PRODUCTS	VEGETABLES & FRUIT
3	1/4
1	1
MILK PRODUCTS	MEAT & ALTERNATIVES

nutrient analysis

PER SERVING			
Calories	532	Carbohydrate	67 g
Protein	29.6 g	Dietary Fiber	4.0 g
Fat	15.2 g	Sodium	660 mg

Excellent source of
thiamin, riboflavin,
niacin, folacin, vitamin
B$_{12}$, calcium, iron and
zinc. **Good** source of
vitamin A. **High** in
dietary fiber.

SERVES 4

Reneé Crompton, RD
OTTAWA, ON

Pasta with Roasted Vegetables and Goat Cheese

4 cups	cubed zucchini	1 L
2 cups	cubed eggplant	500 mL
2 cups	roughly chopped red bell peppers	500 mL
1 cup	roughly chopped sweet white or red onions	250 mL
2 tbsp	olive oil	25 mL
1 1/2 tsp	dried Italian seasoning or French herbs	7 mL
3 1/2 to 4 oz	goat cheese, crumbled	100 to 125 g
8 oz	rotini, penne or other pasta	250 g
	Parmesan cheese (optional)	

TIP

This dish is a great way to increase your vegetable intake. Prepare the recipe with the ingredients as given here or with any other vegetables that your family likes. If there are any leftovers, they're delicious served cold or reheated for lunch the next day.

For best flavor, use fresh herbs rather than dried, but add them at the very end with the cheese. Use about 2 tbsp (25 mL) fresh for every 1 tsp (5 mL) dried.

Nutrition Facts

When choosing vegetables for roasting, go for those with darker colors of red, orange and green; they are richest in nutrients and phytochemicals.

Make Ahead

Vegetables can be roasted up to one day in advance. Reheat in a hot oven for 5 to 10 minutes or until piping hot.

Variation

This vegetable mixture is equally spectacular on a pizza crust covered with a thin layer of pesto or pizza sauce.

1. Put zucchini, eggplant, peppers and onions in a large bowl. Add oil and herbs; toss to coat. Place vegetables in a single layer on prepared baking sheet; roast, stirring occasionally, for 30 to 40 minutes or until vegetables are golden and slightly softened.

2. Meanwhile, in a pot of boiling water, cook pasta according to package directions or until tender but firm; drain.

3. Toss vegetables with pasta. Crumble goat cheese over top; toss to combine or leave as is and sprinkle with Parmesan cheese, if desired.

Complete the meal

This dish is wonderful for casual entertaining. Finish the meal with ORANGE CRÈME CARAMEL (see recipe, page 168).

food guide servings

GRAIN PRODUCTS	VEGETABLES & FRUIT
2	4 1/2
1/2	
MILK PRODUCTS	MEAT & ALTERNATIVES

nutrient analysis

PER SERVING			
Calories	395	Carbohydrate	56.3 g
Protein	13.7 g	Dietary Fiber	6.5 g
Fat	13.4 g	Sodium	99 mg

Excellent source of iron, vitamin C, vitamin A, thiamin, riboflavin, niacin and folacin. **Good** source of zinc and vitamin B$_6$. **Very high** in dietary fiber.

SERVES 8

Piquant Tomato Sauce

Laurie A. Wadsworth, PDt
ANTIGONISH, NS

P

MAKES 7 CUPS (1.75 L)

While bottled or canned pasta sauces are convenient, they don't match the flavor of homemade.

This sauce is based on an old family recipe. It's thick, rich and spicy – ideal for serving with pasta. Even better, the sauce is lower in sodium than commercially prepared sauces. It also freezes well.

2 tbsp	olive oil or vegetable oil	25 mL
1 cup	chopped onions	250 mL
2 tsp	minced garlic	10 mL
1	can (28 oz [798 mL]) diced tomatoes	1
1	can (14 oz [398 mL]) tomato paste, plus one can of water	1
2 tsp	brown sugar	10 mL
1 to 2 tsp	crushed red pepper flakes	5 to 10 mL
	Black pepper to taste	

1. In a large saucepan or Dutch oven, heat oil over medium heat. Add onions and garlic; cook for 4 to 5 minutes or until onions are translucent. Do not allow garlic to brown.

2. Add tomatoes and tomato paste. Fill tomato paste can with water and stir to incorporate any remaining paste; add to tomato mixture along with sugar and red pepper flakes. Cover and bring to a boil. Reduce heat and simmer for 2 hours, stirring occasionally. Season to taste with pepper.

TIP

For a smoother sauce, substitute canned crushed tomatoes for the diced tomatoes.

To serve 8 people, use 1 lb (500 g) dry pasta.

Complete the meal

Add meat to the sauce and serve over pasta sprinkled with Parmesan cheese.

food guide servings

GRAIN PRODUCTS	VEGETABLES & FRUIT
	3
MILK PRODUCTS	MEAT & ALTERNATIVES

nutrient analysis

PER SERVING			
Calories	110	Carbohydrate	17.9 g
Protein	3.3 g	Dietary Fiber	3.7 g
Fat	4.2 g	Sodium	202 mg

Excellent source of vitamin C. **Good** source of vitamin A, iron and vitamin B_6. **Moderate** source of dietary fiber.

SERVES 4

Laurie A. Wadsworth, PDt
ANTIGONISH, NS

Penne with Mushrooms and Spicy Tomato Sauce

TIP

Use any combination of fresh or dried reconstituted mushrooms to make this yummy sauce. Just be sure that most of the moisture has evaporated before adding the rest of the ingredients.

If using dried mushrooms:
Place mushrooms in a bowl; add enough water to cover by about 1 inch (2.5 cm). Let soak for about 30 minutes; drain. Strain soaking liquid through cheesecloth to remove any grit and use it as a flavoring for soups. Trim stems, slice and use as you would fresh mushrooms.

Nutrition Facts
If you use bottled or canned pasta sauce in this recipe, the sodium content will increase to 1102 mg per serving.

8 oz	penne	250 g
1 tbsp	olive oil	15 mL
3 cups	sliced mushrooms	750 mL
1/2 cup	sliced onions	125 mL
1/4 cup	red wine	50 mL
3 cups	PIQUANT TOMATO SAUCE (see recipe, page 150) *or* commercially prepared pasta sauce	750 mL
1/2 tsp	hot pepper sauce	2 mL
2 tbsp	chopped fresh parsley	25 mL
1/4 cup	grated Parmesan cheese	50 mL

1. In a large pot of boiling water, cook pasta until tender but firm; drain.

2. In a large nonstick skillet, heat oil over medium-high heat. Add mushrooms and onions and cook for 6 to 8 minutes or until softened and moisture has evaporated. Add wine and cook, stirring, until evaporated.

3. Stir in PIQUANT TOMATO SAUCE and hot pepper sauce; bring to a boil. Reduce heat and simmer for 1 to 2 minutes. Stir in parsley. Serve over pasta, sprinkled with Parmesan cheese.

complete the meal

Serve with fresh crusty bread and a serving of milk or yogurt.

nutrient analysis

GRAIN PRODUCTS	VEGETABLES & FRUIT
2	3 1/2
1/4	
MILK PRODUCTS	MEAT & ALTERNATIVES

PER SERVING			
Calories	382	Carbohydrate	61.8 g
Protein	13.7 g	Dietary Fiber	6.8 g
Fat	10.1 g	Sodium	297 mg

Excellent source of iron, vitamin C, thiamin, riboflavin, niacin and folacin. **Good** source of zinc, vitamin A and vitamin B$_6$. **Very high** in dietary fiber.

SERVES 4

Rotini with Vegetable Tomato Sauce

Laurie A. Wadsworth, PDt
ANTIGONISH, NS [P]

The simple sauce used here is perfect for those busy weeknight meals and will help boost your vegetable intake.

TIP
For a heartier version of this dish, add 1 cup (250 mL) cooked lentils, or any type of bean and – presto! – you have a protein-rich fagioli or bean sauce.

Nutrition Facts
If you use bottled or canned pasta sauce in this recipe, the sodium content will increase to 1125 mg per serving.

Make Ahead
Make the PIQUANT TOMATO SAUCE ahead of time and freeze in 3-cup (750 mL) portions in airtight containers for up to 3 months.

8 oz	rotini *or* fusilli	250 g
3 cups	PIQUANT TOMATO SAUCE (see recipe, page 150) *or* commercially prepared pasta sauce	750 mL
1 cup	diced zucchini	250 mL
1 cup	shredded carrots	250 mL
1/2 cup	chopped celery	125 mL
2 tbsp	chopped parsley (optional)	25 mL
1/4 cup	grated Parmesan cheese	50 mL

1. In a large pot of boiling water, cook pasta until tender but firm; drain.
2. Meanwhile, in a saucepan over medium-high heat, combine PIQUANT TOMATO SAUCE, zucchini, carrots, celery and parsley; bring to a boil. Reduce heat, cover and simmer for 15 minutes. Serve over pasta. Sprinkle with Parmesan cheese.

Complete the meal
Follow this dish with APRICOT BREAD PUDDING (see recipe, page 158).

food guide servings

GRAIN PRODUCTS	VEGETABLES & FRUIT
2	3 1/2
1/4	
MILK PRODUCTS	MEAT & ALTERNATIVES

nutrient analysis

PER SERVING			
Calories	351	Carbohydrate	62.1 g
Protein	13.1 g	Dietary Fiber	6.9 g
Fat	6.6 g	Sodium	321 mg

Excellent source of iron, vitamin C, vitamin A, thiamin, riboflavin, niacin and folacin. **Good** source of zinc and vitamin B$_6$. **Very high** in dietary fiber.

SERVES 6 — Spinach and Mushroom Pizza Pie

Mary Persi
TORONTO, ON

PREHEAT OVEN TO 375° F (190° C)
12-INCH (30 CM) PIZZA PAN OR BAKING SHEET, GREASED

1 1/2 lbs	prepared pizza dough	750 g
1 tbsp	olive oil	15 mL
2 tsp	minced garlic	10 mL
1/2 cup	chopped onions	125 mL
2 cups	sliced mushrooms	500 mL
1	package (10 oz [300 g]) frozen chopped spinach, thawed and squeezed dry	1
1/8 tsp	nutmeg	0.5 mL
1/4 tsp	black pepper	1 mL
2 cups	grated old Cheddar cheese	500 mL

1. Divide dough into two pieces; one piece (bottom) should be slightly larger than the second (top) piece. Shape the larger piece of dough into a 12-inch (30 cm) circle and place on prepared pizza pan. Set aside.

2. In a large nonstick skillet, heat oil over medium heat. Add garlic, onions and mushrooms; cook, stirring constantly, for 5 to 6 minutes or until mixture is lightly browned. Add spinach and cook, stirring constantly, until all liquid has evaporated and mixture is quite dry. Stir in nutmeg and pepper. Spread mixture evenly over dough; sprinkle with cheese.

3. Roll out top portion of dough and place on top of pizza. Lightly moisten edges and pinch edges together, sealing well. Prick top of pizza all over with a fork. Bake in the bottom half of preheated oven for 25 to 35 minutes or until bottom is browned and top is crispy and golden. Cool for 5 minutes and cut into wedges.

GRAIN PRODUCTS	VEGETABLES & FRUIT
3 1/2	1
3/4	
MILK PRODUCTS	MEAT & ALTERNATIVES

nutrient analysis

PER SERVING			
Calories	496	Carbohydrate	59.2 g
Protein	19.3 g	Dietary Fiber	3.5 g
Fat	20.2 g	Sodium	809 mg

Excellent source of vitamin A, thiamin, riboflavin, niacin, folacin, calcium and iron. **Good** source of vitamin B_{12} and zinc. **Moderate** source of dietary fiber.

SERVES   4

Teriyaki Tofu Stir-Fry

Lorraine Fullum-Bouchard, RD
OTTAWA, ON

"This recipe is great for someone who is trying tofu for the first time," Lorraine says. *"It's easy to prepare and very tasty."*

Variation

Use any vegetables you like, such as broccoli and cauliflower, snow peas and thinly sliced carrots – or any vegetables you have on hand.

Nutrition Facts

Teriyaki sauce is quite high in salt. So if you need to limit your salt intake, replace the teriyaki sauce with sodium-reduced soya sauce.

Complete the meal

Complement this dish with fruit-flavored yogurt for dessert.

1 1/3 cups	diced firm tofu	325 mL
1/2 cup	teriyaki sauce	125 mL
1 tsp	brown sugar	5 mL
1 tsp	cornstarch	5 mL
1 tbsp	water	15 mL
2 tsp	olive oil	10 mL
1/2 cup	diced onions	125 mL
1 cup	diced green bell peppers	250 mL
1 cup	diced red bell peppers	250 mL
1 tsp	minced garlic	5 mL
1 tsp	grated peeled ginger root	5 mL
2 cups	roughly chopped vegetables (see Variation, at left, for suggestions)	500 mL
3 cups	cooked rice	750 mL
1 to 2 tbsp	chopped fresh coriander or parsley (optional)	15 to 25 mL

1. In a medium bowl, gently toss tofu with teriyaki sauce and brown sugar until well coated. Cover and refrigerate for 10 minutes or up to several hours.

2. In a small bowl, whisk together cornstarch and water. Set aside.

3. In a large nonstick skillet, heat oil over medium-high heat. Add onions, green peppers, red peppers, garlic and ginger; stir-fry for 3 minutes. Stir in vegetables of your choice and stir-fry for 3 to 4 minutes or until vegetables are tender-crisp.

4. Add tofu mixture and cornstarch mixture. Stir for 3 to 4 minutes or until thickened and heated through. Serve over rice. Sprinkle with coriander, if using.

food guide servings

GRAIN PRODUCTS	VEGETABLES & FRUIT
1 1/2	2
	1/2
MILK PRODUCTS	MEAT & ALTERNATIVES

nutrient analysis

PER SERVING			
Calories	287	Carbohydrate	49.3 g
Protein	11.9 g	Dietary Fiber	3.0 g
Fat	5.5 g	Sodium	1405 mg

Excellent source of vitamin C and folacin. **Good** source of vitamin A, niacin, vitamin B₆, calcium and iron. **Moderate** source of dietary fiber.

FAST FINISHES

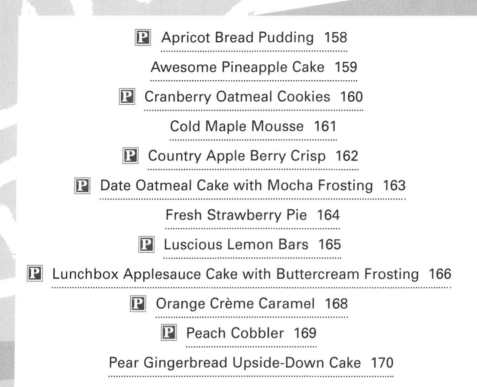

a little 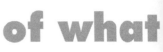 of what

If you love rich desserts, but not all the fat and calories, you don't have to deny yourself completely.

Just eat smaller servings – it's a great way to enjoy the foods you love and control the

are DESSERTS *good for you?*

Here's proof that you can indulge your sweet tooth and still enjoy a healthy diet. In this chapter you'll find a wide variety of family favorites – like cakes, pies, cobblers and crisps. Many of these desserts provide important nutrients, while the rest are just pure indulgence. (And taken in moderation, there's nothing wrong with that!) Of course, all these recipes are fast and easy to make. We've even included lunchbox desserts – to help make your meals away from home more enjoyable.

While desserts and sweets may not be the most nutrient-packed foods in our diet, they taste great and add to our eating enjoyment. And that, in itself, is an important part of good nutrition. Remember, it's not just *what* we eat, but *how* we eat and how we feel. And desserts are an important part of our food traditions and celebrations.

As always, the key is balance. If you are eating well and satisfying your nutrient needs, by all means enjoy a sweet treat now and again.

Think of desserts and sweets as flavorful complements to healthy meals – not as a replacement for more nutrient-rich foods.

If you want to splurge on a rich dessert – such as cake, pie, cheesecake, trifle, crème caramel, pastries or ice cream – just remember to balance the rest of your meal (or meals throughout the day) with lower-fat, more nutritious dishes.

What about "fat-free" desserts?

In order to be called "fat-free," desserts (and other foods) must contain less than 0.5 g fat per serving. But just because something is fat-free doesn't mean that you can eat all you want without gaining weight!

Fat-free foods are best used as part of a well-balanced eating plan. Remember, fat-free doesn't mean calorie-free.

you fancy . . .

amount of calories and fat that you consume. For example, try half a normal serving or one scoop of ice cream instead of two. And if you're eating out, order that rich dessert – and share it!

sweet
suggestions
for kids

Prepare a plate of strawberries, cantaloupe, apples and bananas. Serve with a yogurt dip or chocolate sauce and watch it disappear!

Set out a variety of prepared fruit such as strawberries, grapes, apples, bananas, pears or pineapples. Get out the skewers and let everyone make their own fruit kebabs.

Make ice cream sundaes with sliced bananas, strawberries, canned peaches, pears or mandarin oranges and chocolate or caramel sauce.

Use your blender to make some shakes with fresh fruit and milk, adding ice cream, frozen yogurt or fruit-flavored yogurt.

Tips for HEALTHIER DESSERTS

- **Keep the flavor, but not the fat.** *Try to eat more fruit ices, sorbet, sherbet, frozen yogurt, frozen tofu, ice milk and lower-fat ice cream.*

- **Boost your calcium.** *Good choices include milk pudding, yogurt and rice pudding.*

- **Fill up on fiber.** *Some desserts contain more fiber than others. Try fruit crisps, cobblers and bread puddings.*

- **Be fruitful.** *For refreshing, nutritious desserts, it's hard to beat fresh fruit. Try different combinations, such as melon and grapes, strawberries and pears, melon and blueberries, pears and kiwi, oranges and melon, blueberries and peaches. Have them plain or dress them up with vanilla yogurt, ice cream, frozen yogurt, custard sauce, vanilla pudding or sweetened yogurt cheese. For special occasions, serve fruit, sorbet or sherbet in meringue shells or chocolate cups.*

SERVES 8 — Apricot Bread Pudding

Margie Armstrong
AURORA, ON

P

PREHEAT OVEN TO 350° F (180° C)
10-CUP (2.5 L) SHALLOW BAKING DISH, GREASED

TIP

Any day-old bread works well in this recipe.

Feel free to replace the apricot jam with your favorite fruit preserves.

Nutrition Facts
This recipe represents all four food groups. Nutritious desserts like this one are a great way to complete a meal.

8	slices day-old white bread	8
2 tbsp	butter, softened	25 mL
1/2 cup	apricot jam or other fruit preserves	125 mL
1/2 cup	raisins	125 mL
2 1/2 cups	milk	625 mL
3	eggs	3
1/2 cup	granulated sugar	125 mL
1 tsp	vanilla	5 mL
1 tsp	grated orange zest	5 mL
1/4 tsp	salt	1 mL

1. Spread each bread slice with butter, then apricot jam. Place one slice on top of another to create jam "sandwiches." With a serrated knife, cut into 1-inch (2.5 cm) cubes. Place in baking dish and stir in raisins.

2. In a bowl whisk together milk, eggs, sugar, vanilla, orange zest and salt. Pour over bread cubes. Bake in preheated oven for 50 to 60 minutes or until custard is set in center and top is golden brown.

food guide servings

GRAIN PRODUCTS	VEGETABLES & FRUIT
1	1/2
1/4	1/4
MILK PRODUCTS	MEAT & ALTERNATIVES

nutrient analysis

PER SERVING			
Calories	295	Carbohydrate	51.6 g
Protein	7.8 g	Dietary Fiber	1.0 g
Fat	7.2 g	Sodium	314 mg

Good source of riboflavin and folacin.

SERVES 12 Awesome Pineapple Cake

Zita Bersenas-Cers, RD
HAMILTON, ON

PREHEAT OVEN TO 350° F (180° C)
13- BY 9-INCH (3 L) BAKING PAN, GREASED

"This cake is very quick and easy to make and uses basic ingredients," Zita says. "Children and adults alike love it. It makes a large pan and freezes well."

TIP

One of the things that make this recipe unusual is that it does not use any butter or margarine. Instead, the fat comes from pecans! When you first start mixing the cake, you might think an ingredient is missing because it won't look anything like normal cake batter. But don't worry, it will look just fine when baked.

Nutrition Facts
This dessert is higher in calories and fat, so serve it after a lower-fat meal.

Allergy Alert
Because this cake contains nuts – and a lot of them! – check for nut allergies before serving to guests.

Cake

2 cups	all-purpose flour	500 mL
1 1/2 cups	granulated sugar	375 mL
1 cup	finely chopped pecans	250 mL
1 tsp	baking soda	5 mL
1	can (19 oz [540 mL]) crushed pineapple, with juice	1
2	eggs, beaten	2
1 tsp	vanilla	5 mL

Icing

2 tbsp	butter, softened	25 mL
1	package (4 oz [125 g]) light cream cheese, softened	1
1 1/4 cups	icing sugar	300 mL
1 tsp	vanilla	5 mL

1. Cake: In a large bowl, combine flour, sugar, pecans and baking soda. In another bowl, blend together pineapple, eggs and vanilla. Make a well in the center of dry ingredients and pour in pineapple mixture; stir gently until just combined.

2. Pour batter into prepared pan and bake in preheated oven for 40 to 45 minutes or until a cake tester inserted into the center comes out clean. Set aside to cool.

3. Icing: In a bowl, blend together butter and cream cheese until smooth. Beat in icing sugar and vanilla until smooth. Spread icing over cooled cake.

nutrient analysis

GRAIN PRODUCTS	VEGETABLES & FRUIT
1	1/2
	1/4
MILK PRODUCTS	MEAT & ALTERNATIVES

PER SERVING			
Calories	364	Carbohydrate	61.7 g
Protein	4.9 g	Dietary Fiber	1.7 g
Fat	11.7 g	Sodium	175 mg

Good source of thiamin and folacin.

MAKES 36

Lynn Roblin, RD   P

Cranberry Oatmeal Cookies

PREHEAT OVEN TO 350° F (180° C)
BAKING SHEETS, GREASED

These cookies are quick to make, fun to eat and they're so easy that Bev's 10-year-old daughter Lisa can make them on her own.

TIP

Here's a tip from Ruby Bruce of South Lake, PEI: If you're looking for a supply of freshly baked cookies, make up a batch of your favorite cookie dough and bake some of your favorite cookies for immediate enjoyment. Form remaining cookie dough into small balls, place on cookie sheets and freeze. When frozen, put into a container and store in the freezer. Whenever you want a dozen freshly baked cookies, remove cookie balls from freezer, let thaw and bake.

1 cup	all-purpose flour	250 mL
1/4 cup	wheat bran	50 mL
1/2 tsp	baking powder	2 mL
1/2 cup	margarine	125 mL
1/2 cup	granulated sugar	125 mL
1/2 cup	brown sugar	125 mL
1	egg	1
1 tsp	vanilla	5 mL
1 cup	quick-cooking (not instant) oats	250 mL
1/2 cup	dried cranberries	125 mL

1. In a small bowl, combine flour, wheat bran and baking powder. Set aside.

2. In a medium bowl, cream together margarine, granulated sugar and brown sugar until light and fluffy. Add egg and mix well; stir in vanilla. Add flour mixture and blend thoroughly. Stir in oats and cranberries.

3. Drop heaping teaspoons of cookie dough on prepared cookie sheets, about 2 inches (5 cm) apart. Bake in preheated oven for 10 to 12 minutes or until edges are lightly browned.

food guide servings

GRAIN PRODUCTS	VEGETABLES & FRUIT
1/2	

MILK PRODUCTS	MEAT & ALTERNATIVES

nutrient analysis

PER 2 COOKIES			
Calories	147	Carbohydrate	22.8 g
Protein	2.0 g	Dietary Fiber	1.3 g
Fat	5.7 g	Sodium	80 mg

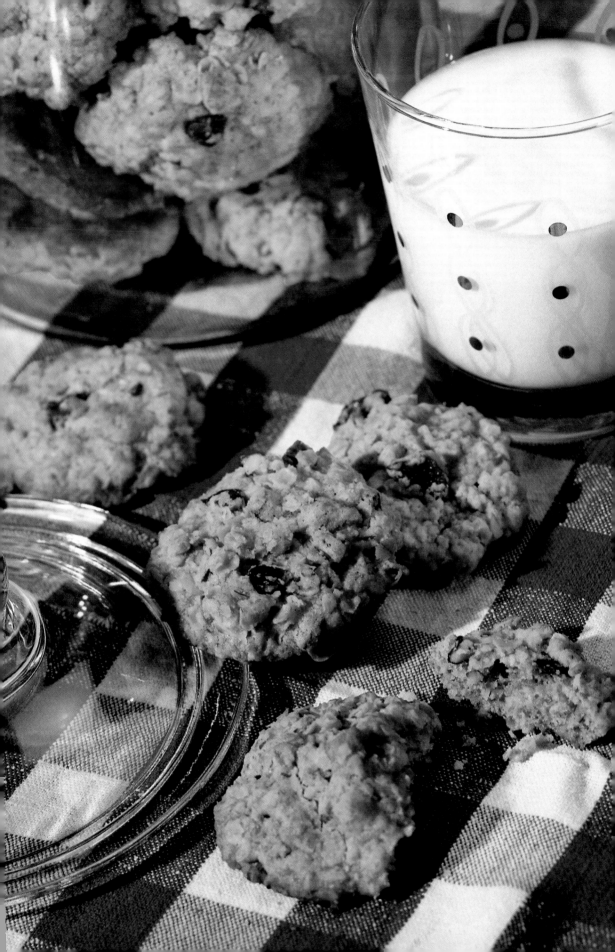

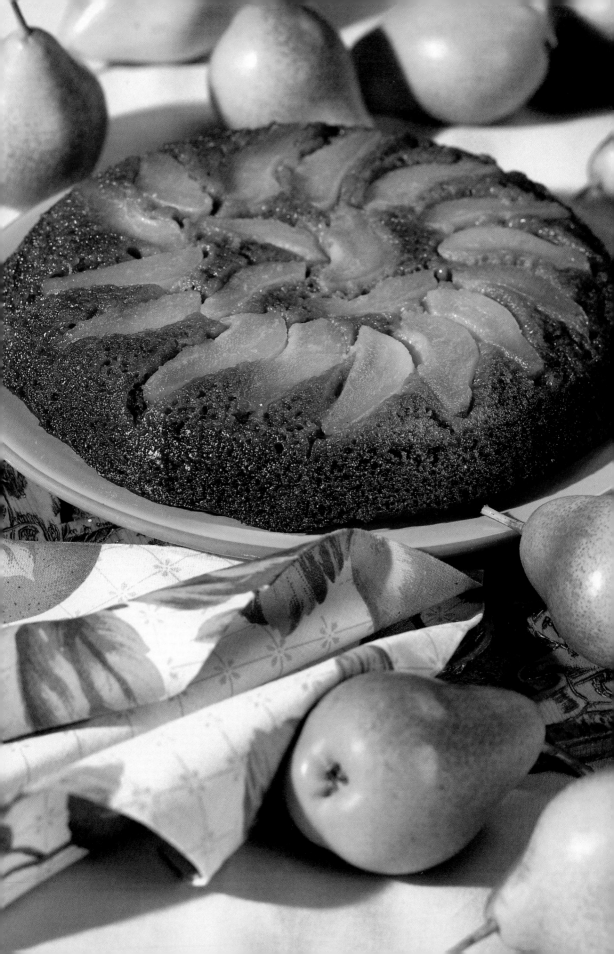

Cold Maple Mousse

Ingrid Ermanovics
MAPLE RIDGE, BC

6-CUP (1.5 L) SOUFFLÉ DISH

A favorite from Ingrid's childhood, this dessert is the one she asked for whenever company came to visit. It's wonderful served with fresh fruit of any kind.

1 tbsp	unflavored gelatin (1 package)	15 mL
2 tbsp	cold water	25 mL
1 cup	maple syrup	250 mL
1	egg, beaten	1
1/8 tsp	salt	0.5 mL
2 cups	whipping (35%) cream	500 mL
1/2 cup	toasted slivered almonds, optional (see Tip, at left)	125 mL

TIP

To toast almonds: In a non-stick skillet over medium heat toast almonds, stirring constantly, for 3 to 4 minutes or until golden brown. Alternatively, microwave on High for 3 to 5 minutes, stirring at 1-minute intervals.

Nutrition Facts

This dessert is an indulgence, so keep your serving size small. It's great to enjoy a small taste and not feel deprived.

1. In a small bowl, soak gelatin in cold water.

2. Meanwhile, in a double boiler over medium-low heat, whisk together maple syrup, egg and salt; cook, stirring constantly, for 5 to 8 minutes or until slightly thickened. Remove from heat and whisk in gelatin. Refrigerate mixture until cool.

3. In a bowl with an electric mixer, whip cream until stiff. Add one-third of the cream to maple mixture; beat until well blended. (This gives the mousse a bit more volume.) Gently fold in the remaining cream. Pour into soufflé dish. Chill until set. Garnish with almonds, if using.

food guide servings

GRAIN PRODUCTS	VEGETABLES & FRUIT

MILK PRODUCTS	MEAT & ALTERNATIVES

nutrient analysis

PER SERVING			
Calories	244	Carbohydrate	21.4 g
Protein	2.4 g	Dietary Fiber	0 g
Fat	17.2 g	Sodium	56 mg

Good source of zinc and vitamin A.

◄ PEAR GINGERBREAD UPSIDE-DOWN CAKE (PAGE 170)

SERVES 4 Country Apple Berry Crisp

Marilynn Small, RD
Post Cereals
Toronto, ON

P

Preheat oven to 375° F (190° C)
4-cup (1 L) baking dish with lid, greased

Nutrition Facts
Packed with fruit and whole grains, each serving of this crisp supplies 2 servings from the Vegetables & Fruit food group, as well as plenty of fiber.

3	large baking apples, cored and thinly sliced	3
2 cups	mixed berries	500 mL
1 tbsp	cornstarch	15 mL
3	large shredded wheat-type biscuits, crumbled	3
1/2 cup	packed brown sugar	125 mL
1/4 cup	butter *or* margarine	50 mL
1 tsp	ground cinnamon	5 mL

1. In a bowl combine apples, berries and cornstarch.
2. In another bowl combine crumbled biscuits, brown sugar, butter and cinnamon. Rub with fingers until crumbly. Set aside 1 cup (250 mL) crumble mixture.
3. Toss remaining crumble mixture with fruit. Place fruit mixture in baking dish. Sprinkle remaining crumb mixture over top.
4. Cover and bake in preheated oven for 20 minutes. Remove cover and bake for 10 minutes or until apples are tender. Serve warm.

food guide servings

Grain Products	Vegetables & Fruit
1/2	2

Milk Products	Meat & Alternatives

nutrient analysis

PER SERVING			
Calories	405	Carbohydrate	75.9 g
Protein	2.7 g	Dietary Fiber	8.6 g
Fat	12.7 g	Sodium	129 mg

Good source of vitamin C. **Very high** in dietary fiber.

SERVES 16

Joan Triandafillou, RD
NEPEAN, ON

P

Date Oatmeal Cake with Mocha Frosting

PREHEAT OVEN TO 350° F (180° C)
9-INCH (2.5 L) SQUARE BAKING PAN, GREASED

Nutrition Facts
The calories and fat in this dessert are a little higher than average, so choose a smaller serving size or balance it with a lighter main meal.

Allergy Alert
Check for nut allergies before serving this cake to guests. It doesn't contain eggs, however, so people with egg allergies may be able to enjoy it.

Cake

1 cup	rolled oats	250 mL
1 1/2 cups	boiling water	375 mL
1 cup	all-purpose flour	250 mL
1 tsp	baking soda	5 mL
1/4 tsp	salt	1 mL
1/2 cup	margarine	125 mL
1 cup	brown sugar	250 mL
1 tsp	vanilla	5 mL
1 cup	chopped dates	250 mL
1/2 cup	chopped walnuts	125 mL

Mocha Frosting

2 tbsp	margarine	25 mL
1 1/4 cups	sifted icing sugar	300 mL
2 tsp	cocoa powder	10 mL
1 tbsp	strong coffee, cooled	15 mL
1 tsp	vanilla	5 mL

1. Cake: In a small bowl, combine oats and boiling water; let stand until cool.

2. In a separate bowl, combine flour, baking soda and salt. Set aside.

3. In a large bowl, cream together margarine and brown sugar until fluffy. Beat in vanilla, rolled-oats mixture and flour mixture. Stir in dates and walnuts. Pour mixture into prepared pan and bake in preheated oven for 30 to 35 minutes or until cake tester inserted into center comes out clean. Set aside to cool.

4. Mocha Frosting: In a bowl, blend together margarine, sugar, cocoa, coffee and vanilla until fluffy. If necessary, thin icing with extra coffee to reach desired consistency. Spread over cooled cake.

nutrient analysis

GRAIN PRODUCTS	VEGETABLES & FRUIT
1/2	1/2
MILK PRODUCTS	MEAT & ALTERNATIVES

PER SERVING			
Calories	252	Carbohydrate	40.0 g
Protein	2.5 g	Dietary Fiber	2.1 g
Fat	10.0 g	Sodium	211 mg

Moderate source of dietary fiber.

SERVES 6   Fresh Strawberry Pie

Meredith Jackson, RD
OAKVILLE, ON

Enjoy this simply delicious pie when fresh strawberries are in season. Use it as an excuse to get out to pick your own berries – it's a great family activity!

Nutrition Facts
Strawberries are an excellent source of vitamin C. Use them fresh or frozen, not only for desserts, but with pancakes, cereal, yogurt or salads.

4 cups	hulled strawberries	1 L
1/3 cup	cold water	75 mL
1/4 cup	granulated sugar	50 mL
4 tsp	cornstarch, mixed with 2 tbsp (25 mL) water	20 mL
1	prepared 9-inch (22.5 cm) graham cracker crumb crust	1
1 cup	whipped cream (optional) *or* Whipped Cream and Yogurt Topping (see recipe, page 171)	250 mL

1. Purée or mash 1 cup (250 mL) of the strawberries. You should have about 3/4 cup (175 mL) puréed berries.

2. In a small saucepan, combine puréed strawberries, water and sugar; blend well. Bring to a boil over medium heat; whisk in cornstarch mixture. Cook, stirring constantly, for 1 minute or until slightly thickened. Remove from heat and allow to cool slightly.

3. Place remaining berries, stem-end down, in pie shell. Spoon purée mixture evenly over berries. Chill until glaze is set, about 3 hours.

4. Serve alone or, if desired, with whipped cream or Whipped Cream and Yogurt Topping.

food guide servings

GRAIN PRODUCTS	VEGETABLES & FRUIT
1/4	1

MILK PRODUCTS	MEAT & ALTERNATIVES

nutrient analysis

PER SERVING			
Calories	196	Carbohydrate	34.5 g
Protein	2.0 g	Dietary Fiber	2.5 g
Fat	6.8 g	Sodium	178 mg

Excellent source of vitamin C. **Moderate** source of fiber.

Dairy Farmers of Canada

MAKES 15 — Luscious Lemon Bars

P

PREHEAT OVEN TO 350° F (180° C)
8-INCH (2 L) SQUARE BAKING PAN

We all need to sit back and relax every once in a while. So take a break and enjoy one of these lemon bars with a quiet cup of tea.

Nutrition Facts
These bars are less about nutrition than pure eating pleasure. But don't worry – a little indulgence, practised in moderation, is still an important part of healthy, balanced eating.

1 1/3 cups	all-purpose flour	325 mL
1 cup	granulated sugar	250 mL
1/2 cup	butter, softened	125 mL
2	eggs	2
2 tbsp	all-purpose flour	25 mL
1/4 tsp	baking powder	1 mL
1 1/2 tsp	grated lemon zest	7 mL
3 tbsp	lemon juice	45 mL
	Icing sugar	

1. In a medium bowl, blend together 1 1/3 cups (325 mL) flour, 1/4 cup (50 mL) of the granulated sugar and butter until mixture is crumbly. Press into bottom of baking pan. Bake in preheated oven for 15 minutes or until edges are lightly browned.

2. In a small bowl, beat together remaining granulated sugar, eggs, 2 tbsp (25 mL) flour, baking powder, lemon zest and lemon juice. Pour filling over hot crust. Bake for 15 minutes or until filling is set. Cool in pan on wire rack. Sprinkle with icing sugar. Cut into bars.

nutrient analysis

GRAIN PRODUCTS	VEGETABLES & FRUIT
1/2	
MILK PRODUCTS	MEAT & ALTERNATIVES

PER SERVING			
Calories	161	Carbohydrate	22.9 g
Protein	2.2 g	Dietary Fiber	0.4 g
Fat	6.9 g	Sodium	76 mg

SERVES 9

Marguerite McDuff
ST LOUIS DE BLANDFORD, PQ P

Lunchbox Applesauce Cake with Buttercream Frosting

PREHEAT OVEN TO 350° F (180° C)
8-INCH (2 L) SQUARE BAKING PAN, GREASED

Pack pieces of this moist and delicious cake in lunch bags and wait for the raves at the end of the day. But don't limit this treat to the brown baggers – it's delicious anytime!

Variation

It's easy to turn this recipe into pumpkin or banana cake. Just substitute 1 cup (250 mL) pumpkin purée or mashed ripe bananas (about 2 medium) for 3/4 cup (175 mL) the applesauce.

Allergy Alert

For people who are lactose-intolerant or have milk allergies, just replace the frosting with a mixture of icing sugar and cinnamon sprinkled over the cake.

Cake

1 1/2 cups	all-purpose flour	375 mL
1 tsp	baking powder	5 mL
1 tsp	ground cinnamon	5 mL
1/2 tsp	salt	2 mL
1/2 tsp	baking soda	2 mL
1/4 tsp	ground nutmeg	1 mL
1/4 tsp	ground cloves	1 mL
2	eggs	2
1/4 cup	vegetable oil	50 mL
1/3 cup	granulated sugar	75 mL
1/3 cup	packed brown sugar	75 mL
3/4 cup	applesauce	175 mL

Frosting

2 tbsp	butter, softened	25 mL
1 cup	sifted icing sugar	250 mL
1 tbsp	milk *or* cream	15 mL
1/2 tsp	vanilla	2 mL

1. **Cake:** In a bowl sift together flour, baking powder, cinnamon, salt, baking soda, nutmeg and cloves. Set aside.

2. In a large bowl with an electric mixer, blend eggs, oil, granulated sugar and brown sugar at high speed for 1 minute or until mixture is light and fluffy. Stir in applesauce; blend at medium speed for 30 seconds. Add dry ingredients; blend at medium speed for 30 seconds or until well combined. Pour into prepared pan and bake in preheated oven for 35 to 40 minutes or until a cake tester inserted in the center comes out clean. Cool in pan.

3. Frosting: In a medium bowl with an electric mixer, blend butter, icing sugar, milk and vanilla at high speed for 2 minutes or until light and creamy. Add additional milk as required to reach desired spreading consistency. Spread frosting on top of cake. Sprinkle with cinnamon.

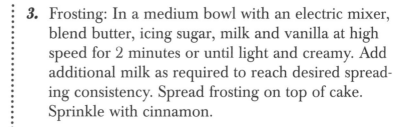

nutrient analysis

GRAIN PRODUCTS	VEGETABLES & FRUIT
1	
MILK PRODUCTS	MEAT & ALTERNATIVES

PER SERVING			
Calories	288	Carbohydrate	46.7 g
Protein	3.7 g	Dietary Fiber	1.0 g
Fat	10.0 g	Sodium	266 mg

SERVES 8 — Orange Crème Caramel

*Canadian Egg
Marketing Agency*   P

PREHEAT OVEN TO 350° F (180° C)
8-INCH (2 L) ROUND BAKING PAN

Here's the perfect finish for a special meal with family or friends.

Nutrition Facts

This recipe is a lighter, but even tastier, variation of traditional crème caramel. It makes a nice balance to a heavier main course.

Make Ahead

Prepare up to 2 days ahead. Cover with foil or plastic wrap and refrigerate.

1/2 cup	granulated sugar	125 mL
1/4 cup	water	50 mL
5	eggs	5
1/2 cup	granulated sugar	125 mL
2 1/2 cups	hot milk	625 mL
1 tbsp	grated orange zest	15 mL
1 tsp	vanilla extract	5 mL

1. In a small heavy saucepan, combine 1/2 cup (125 mL) sugar and water. Cook over medium heat, stirring constantly, until sugar is dissolved. (Be careful not to let the mixture boil at this stage.) Increase heat to medium-high and boil, without stirring, for 6 to 8 minutes or until mixture caramelizes and is golden in color. Pour immediately into pan, tilting pan to cover bottom.

2. In a medium bowl, stir together eggs and 1/2 cup (125 mL) sugar until blended. Stir in hot milk, orange zest and vanilla; avoid overmixing. Pour into pan over caramel mixture. Place baking pan in a larger pan of boiling water. Bake in preheated oven for 40 to 45 minutes or until mixture is set. Remove from hot water. Cool on a rack. Refrigerate until ready to serve.

3. To remove from pan, run a spatula carefully around custard. Invert a rimmed serving plate over custard and turn over. Serve in wedges with caramel sauce from the pan.

food guide servings

GRAIN PRODUCTS	VEGETABLES & FRUIT
1/4	1/2
MILK PRODUCTS	MEAT & ALTERNATIVES

nutrient analysis

PER SERVING			
Calories	183	Carbohydrate	29.2 g
Protein	6.4 g	Dietary Fiber	0.1 g
Fat	4.6 g	Sodium	78 mg

Good source of riboflavin and vitamin B$_{12}$.

Margie Armstrong
AURORA, ON [P]

SERVES 6

Peach Cobbler

PREHEAT OVEN TO 350° F (180° C)
8-INCH (2 L) BAKING DISH, GREASED

Prepare this easy-to-make cobbler and let it bake in the oven while you are eating dinner. Enjoy while still warm, served with vanilla ice cream or frozen yogurt.

TIP

When fresh peaches are in season use 3 cups (750 mL) peeled sliced peaches and omit the canned peaches and juice. Stir the peaches up a bit (to release some juices) and sprinkle the sugar/cornstarch mixture over them. Add the lemon juice and stir to blend.

Nutrition Facts

Choose desserts like this one when you need to add to your daily servings of grains and fruit.

Filling

1	can (28 oz [796 mL]) sliced peaches, drained, reserving 1/2 cup (125 mL) juice	1
2 tbsp	granulated sugar	25 mL
2 tsp	cornstarch	10 mL
1 tsp	lemon juice	5 mL

Topping

1 cup	biscuit baking mix	250 mL
1/8 tsp	nutmeg	0.5 mL
1/3 cup	milk	75 mL

1. **Filling:** Place peaches in prepared baking dish. In a bowl combine sugar and cornstarch; whisk in reserved peach juice. Stir in lemon juice. Pour mixture over peaches. Set aside.

2. **Topping:** In a medium bowl, combine baking mix and nutmeg; stir in milk to form a sticky dough. Drop dough by the tablespoon on top of the peach mixture. (Not all of the filling will be covered.) Bake in preheated oven for 40 to 45 minutes or until crust is lightly browned.

GRAIN PRODUCTS	VEGETABLES & FRUIT
1	1
MILK PRODUCTS	MEAT & ALTERNATIVES

nutrient analysis

PER SERVING			
Calories	158	Carbohydrate	31.6 g
Protein	2.7 g	Dietary Fiber	1.4 g
Fat	2.8 g	Sodium	272 mg

SERVES 12

Barbara Selley, RD
TORONTO, ON

Pear Gingerbread Upside-Down Cake

PREHEAT OVEN TO 350° F (180° C)
9-INCH (2.5 L) SQUARE BAKING PAN, GREASED

This dessert is delicious on its own, but for a little extra decadence, serve it with Whipped Cream and Yogurt Topping (see recipe, facing page.) Don't overdo it, however, or you'll add too many calories and too much fat to your dessert.

Nutrition Facts
The molasses in this cake makes it a good source of iron.

Topping

1/4 cup	butter, melted	50 mL
1/2 cup	packed brown sugar	125 mL
1	can (28 oz [796 mL]) pear halves, drained	1

Cake

1/4 cup	butter, softened	50 mL
1/2 cup	packed brown sugar	125 mL
2	eggs	2
1 cup	applesauce	250 mL
1/2 cup	fancy molasses	125 mL
1 1/2 cups	all-purpose flour	375 mL
2 tsp	ground ginger	10 mL
1 tsp	baking powder	5 mL
1 tsp	baking soda	5 mL
1 tsp	ground cinnamon	5 mL
1/2 tsp	ground cloves	2 mL
1/4 tsp	salt	1 mL

1. Topping: In a bowl combine melted butter and brown sugar; spread in the bottom of baking pan. Lay pears on top of sugar, cut-side up. Slice any large pieces in half.

2. Cake: In a large bowl using an electric mixer, cream together butter and brown sugar. Add eggs and beat until light and fluffy. Blend in applesauce and molasses.

3. In a separate bowl, combine flour, ginger, baking powder, baking soda, cinnamon, cloves and salt. Stir into applesauce mixture.

4. Spoon batter over pear topping. Bake in preheated oven for 45 to 50 minutes or until a cake tester inserted into center comes out clean.

5. Run a knife around the edges of the cake and immediately invert onto a serving platter. Leave the pan on top of the inverted cake for 1 to 2 minutes to allow all of the topping to drip onto cake.

Whipped Cream and Yogurt Topping

This is Barbara Selley's multipurpose dessert topping: Beat 1/2 cup (125 mL) whipping cream until thick; add 1 tbsp (15 mL) sugar and 1/2 tsp (2 mL) vanilla. Whip cream until stiff. Gently fold in 1/2 cup (125 mL) plain lower-fat yogurt until thoroughly combined. Makes 1 1/2 cups (375 mL).

Contains 88 calories and 7.4 g fat per 1/4-cup (50 mL) serving: the same amount of regular whipped cream provides 103 calories and 11 g fat – and less calcium.

GRAIN PRODUCTS	VEGETABLES & FRUIT
1/2	1/2
MILK PRODUCTS	MEAT & ALTERNATIVES

nutrient analysis

PER SERVING			
Calories	279	Carbohydrate	48.6 g
Protein	3.0 g	Dietary Fiber	1.7 g
Fat	8.8 g	Sodium	266 mg

Good source of iron.

SUNDAY	MONDAY	TUESDAY	WEDNESDAY
Eat Together Night	**Make and Bake Night**	**Super Easy**	**One-Dish Wonder**
BAKED CHICKEN AND POTATO DINNER	VEGGIE, BEEF AND PASTA BAKE	PARMESAN-HERB BAKED FISH FILLETS	SKILLET PORK CHOPS WITH SWEET POTATOES AND COUSCOUS
or	or	or	or
PORK TENDERLOIN WITH ROASTED POTATOES	TURKEY POT PIE	EXOTIC GINGER-CUMIN CHICKEN	CHICKPEA HOT POT Whole grain rolls
•	or	•	—
Green beans	PASTITSIO	Quick Microwave Rice	Sherbet
HONEY-GLAZED CARROTS	FAST AND EASY GREEK SALAD	Steamed broccoli	
Whole grain rolls		—	
—	*Tip: All can be made*	Fruit-flavored yogurt	
COUNTRY APPLE BERRY CRISP	*ahead on Sunday*		
		Tip: Make extra rice if having	
		HURRY-UP FILL-ME-UP	
		BURRITOS on Thursday	
The Gang's All Here	**Made Ahead**	**Soup Night**	**Noodle Night**
BROILED HAM STEAK WITH PINEAPPLE-MANGO SALSA	SPAGHETTINI WITH TUNA AND OLIVES	BEEF, VEGETABLE AND BEAN SOUP	FETTUCCINE CARBONARA
EASY SCALLOPED POTATOES	or	or	or
Steamed green vegetables	ROTINI WITH VEGETABLE TOMATO SAUCE	SEAFOOD CHOWDER	CREAMY PASTA AND BROCCOLI
or	—	or	or
SALISBURY STEAK IN WINE SAUCE	Frozen yogurt	CHUNKY VEGETABLE LENTIL SOUP	CHINESE ALMOND CHICKEN WITH NOODLES
Mashed potatoes		•	•
Peas	*Tip: Use rest of PIQUANT*	Whole grain bread	Bagged salad
Whole grain bread	*TOMATO SAUCE prepared*		Dressing
—	*on Saturday*	*Tip: Can make soup ahead*	
LUSCIOUS LEMON BARS		*on weekend*	
Picnic Lunch/Supper	**Really Easy**	**Salad Supper**	**Fast Fix**
Cold chicken	QUICK STEAMED FISH FILLETS WITH POTATOES AND ASPARAGUS	SALMON, POTATO AND GREEN BEAN SALAD	HOISIN BEEF AND BROCCOLI STIR-FRY
or	or	or	or
Lean deli meats	TUNA SALAD MELTS	CHICKEN AND BEAN SALAD	PORK CHOPS WITH PEACHES AND KIWI
•	Raw vegetables	or	or
GERMAN POTATO SALAD PICNIC-STYLE	HONEY-MUSTARD DIP	FAST AND EASY GREEK SALAD	TERIYAKI TOFU STIR-FRY
•	or	•	•
BEET, ORANGE AND JICAMA SALAD	TOMATO AND BEAN SOUP	Pita bread	Quick Microwave Rice
•	Whole wheat toast, rolls or bagels		
Fresh rolls		*Tip: Purchase cooked*	*Tip: Make extra rice for Friday*
—		*chicken at deli*	
Chocolate Cake			
•			
Watermelon			

THURSDAY	FRIDAY	SATURDAY
Kids in the Kitchen	**Friday Night Supper**	**Make Ahead**
HURRY-UP FILL-ME-UP BURRITOS	RED PEPPER AND GOAT CHEESE PIZZA	PIQUANT TOMATO SAUCE
or	or	•
FAVORITE CHICKEN FAJITAS	SPINACH AND MUSHROOM PIZZA PIE	PENNE WITH MUSHROOMS AND SPICY TOMATO SAUCE
—	—	*Tip: Save half the sauce for Tuesday*
Fresh or canned fruit Vanilla pudding	Frozen yogurt	•
	•	French or Italian bread
	CRANBERRY OATMEAL COOKIES	•
Tip: Kids under 10 need		Bagged salad Dressing
adult supervision		—
		LUNCHBOX APPLESAUCE CAKE
Make Ahead/Fast Fix	**Crowd Pleaser**	**Special Night**
CREOLE CROCKPOT CHICKEN	FAST CHILI	SALMON WITH ROASTED VEGETABLES
Quick Microwave Rice	or	Brown rice
or	CROWD-PLEASING VEGETARIAN CHILI	or
TUNA AND RICE CASSEROLE	or	CURRIED RED PEPPER CHICKEN
or	STICKY HONEY GARLIC CHICKEN WINGS	Coconut Rice
SWISS CHARD FRITTATA IN A PITA	•	CUCUMBER RAITA SALAD
	Quick Microwave Rice	—
		Fresh fruit
	Raw vegetables HERBED YOGURT DIP	or
	•	PEACH COBBLER
	Garlic toasts	
	—	
	Sherbet	
On the Grill	**Planned Over**	**Patio Party**
HOT 'N' SPICY TURKEY BURGERS	EGG AND MUSHROOM FRIED RICE	Pita crisps Raw vegetables
or	or	FIERY VERDE DIP
ASIAN FLANK STEAK	BAKED CHICKEN PARMESAN	•
or	Quick Microwave Rice	BARBECUED BEEF SATAYS
CRUNCHY FISH BURGERS	•	•
•	Green vegetable	COLORFUL BEAN AND CORN SALAD
QUICK MARINATED BEAN SALAD	*Tip: Use rice from Wednesday*	CREAMY BROCCOLI SALAD
or		•
SWEET POTATO "FRIES"		Bread basket
—		—
Ice cream cones		FRESH STRAWBERRY PIE
		or
		Angel food cake with berries and Whipped Cream and Yogurt topping

How Long Will It Keep?

These are general guidelines for the shelf-life of common foods. Read the label and check "best before" dates, if applicable. Once opened, the best before date no longer applies. Some foods are safe to eat if stored longer, but flavor and nutritive value will deteriorate. Discard foods if there is evidence of spoilage.

	REFRIGERATOR	FREEZER
Casseroles, meat pies, meat sauces, cooked	2 to 3 days	3 months
Cheese, firm	several months	3 months
Cheese, processed		
Unopened	several months	
Opened	3 to 4 weeks	3 months
Eggs	3 weeks	
Fish, cooked	1 to 2 days	
Fish, raw		
Higher-fat species (salmon, mackerel, lake trout)	1 to 2 days	2 months
Lower-fat species (cod, haddock, pike, smelt)	1 to 2 days	6 months
Meat, all, cooked	3 to 4 days	2 to 3 months
Meat, cold cuts, opened	3 to 4 days	
Meat, cured or smoked	6 to 7 days	1 to 2 months
Meat, ground, raw	1 to 2 days	2 to 3 months
Meat, roasts, raw	3 to 4 days	10 to 12 months
Meat, steaks and chops, raw	2 to 3 days	8 to 12 months
Milk, cream, cottage cheese, yogurt, opened	3 days	
Poultry, cooked	3 to 4 days	1 to 3 months
Poultry, raw		
Pieces	2 to 3 days	6 months
Whole	2 to 3 days	1 year
Salad dressings and mayonnaise		
Opened	1 to 2 months	
Scallops, shrimp, raw	1 to 2 days	2 to 4 months
Shellfish, cooked	1 to 2 days	
Soups	2 to 3 days	4 months

*Adapted from the Ontario Ministry of Agriculture, Food and Rural Affairs, Food Handlers' Storage Guide (dated 1995).

Canadian Guidelines for Healthy Weights
Body Mass Index (BMI)

for adults 20-65 years of age

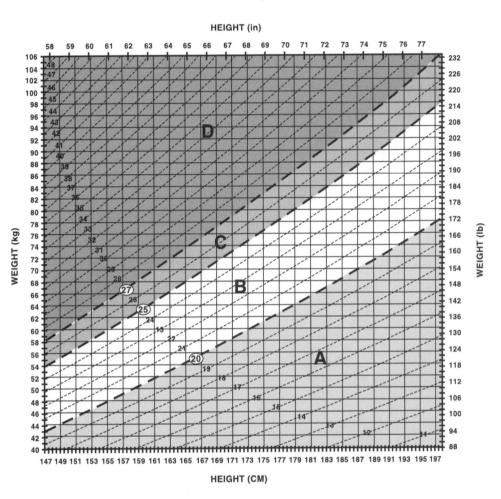

To estimate BMI, locate the point on the chart where height and weight intersect. Read the number on the dashed line closest to this point. For example, if you weigh 69 kg and are 173 cm tall, you have a BMI of approximately 23, which is in Zone B.

You can also calculate your BMI using this formula: $BMI = \dfrac{weight\ (kg)}{height\ (m^2)}$

Zone	BMI	Health Effects
A	< 20	May be associated with health problems for some people
B	20 - 25	Good weight for most people
C	25 - 27	May lead to health problems in some people
D	>27	Increased risk of developing health problems

Source: Health and Welfare Canada. Promoting Healthy Weights: A Discussion Paper. Minister of Supply and Services Canada: Ottawa, Ontario. 1988

Health   Santé
Canada   Canada

Canadä

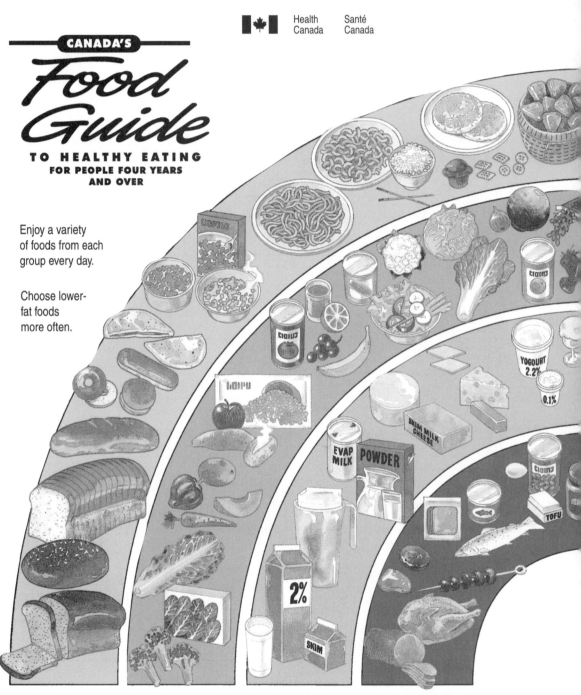

CANADA'S
Food
Guide

TO HEALTHY EATING
FOR PEOPLE FOUR YEARS
AND OVER

Health Canada   Santé Canada

Enjoy a variety
of foods from each
group every day.

Choose lower-
fat foods
more often.

Grain Products
Choose whole grain
and enriched products
more often.

Vegetables and Fruit
Choose dark green and
orange vegetables and
orange fruit more often.

Milk Products
Choose lower-fat milk
products more often.

Meat and Alternatives
Choose leaner meats,
poultry and fish, as well
as dried peas, beans
and lentils more often.

Canada

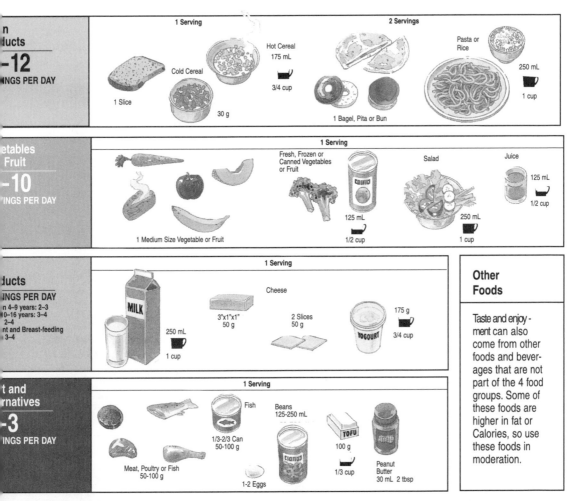

n
ducts

-12
INGS PER DAY

1 Serving		2 Servings	
1 Slice	Cold Cereal 30 g	Hot Cereal 175 mL 3/4 cup	Pasta or Rice 250 mL 1 cup
		1 Bagel, Pita or Bun	

etables
Fruit

-10
INGS PER DAY

1 Serving			
1 Medium Size Vegetable or Fruit	Fresh, Frozen or Canned Vegetables or Fruit 125 mL 1/2 cup	Salad 250 mL 1 cup	Juice 125 mL 1/2 cup

ducts

INGS PER DAY
n 4–9 years: 2–3
0–16 years: 3–4
2–4
nt and Breast-feeding
3–4

1 Serving			
MILK 250 mL 1 cup	Cheese 3"x1"x1" 50 g	2 Slices 50 g	YOGOURT 175 g 3/4 cup

t and
rnatives

-3
INGS PER DAY

1 Serving			
Meat, Poultry or Fish 50-100 g	Fish 1/3-2/3 Can 50-100 g	1-2 Eggs	Beans 125-250 mL 1/3 cup	TOFU 100 g	Peanut Butter 30 mL 2 tbsp

Other Foods

Taste and enjoy - ment can also come from other foods and beverages that are not part of the 4 food groups. Some of these foods are higher in fat or Calories, so use these foods in moderation.

ent People Need Different Amounts of Food

mount of food you need every day from the 4 food groups and other foods depends on your age, body size, activity level, er you are male or female and if you are pregnant or breast-feeding. That's why the Food Guide gives a lower and higher er of servings for each food group. For example, young children can choose the lower number of servings, while male gers can go to the higher number. Most other people can choose servings somewhere in between.

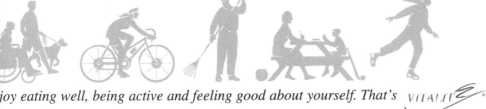

joy eating well, being active and feeling good about yourself. That's VITALITÉ

Canadian Diabetes Association

Food Choice System

The Canadian Diabetes Association Food Choice Values have been assigned to the recipes in this book in accordance with the Good Health Eating Guide (1994) which is used for meal planning by people with diabetes. The Food Choice Values for a certain serving size have been calculated for each recipe to make it easy to fit into an individualized meal plan. (Food Choice Value calculations do not include optional ingredients.) Servings must be carefully measured, since changing the serving size will increase or decrease the Food Choice Value assigned. Some recipes may include an inappropriate portion of a certain food choice for the person with diabetes. With these recipes, it is recommended that the portion be reduced to help include the recipe in the meal plan.

The Canadian Diabetes Association Food Choice System used in the Good Health Eating Guide (1994) is based on *Canada's Food Guide to Healthy Eating.* For more information on diabetes contact the Canadian Diabetes Association National Office:
15 Toronto Street, Suite 800, Toronto, Ontario M5C 2E3
E-mail: info@cda-nat.org
Internet: http://www.diabetes.ca

GETTING OFF TO A GREAT START — FOOD CHOICE PER SERVING

PAGE	RECIPE	SERVING SIZE	■	●	◆	✳	◉	▲	++
30	Sunny Orange Shake (1% milk choice)	1		1	3	2 1/2			
31	Banana-Berry Wake-Up Shake (2% milk choice)	1/2 recipe		1 1/2	2	1 1/2			
32	Banana Bread	1/12 recipe	1	1/2			1/2	1	
33	Big-Batch Bran Muffins	1 muffin	2	1/2			1 1/2	2	
34	Cornmeal Muffins	1 muffin	1 1/2				1	1	
35	Pumpkin Raisin Muffins	1 muffin	1	1			1/2	1	
36	Orange-Apricot Oatmeal Scones	1 scone	1 1/2				1/2	1 1/2	
37	Creamy Microwave Oatmeal (2% milk choice)	1	1 1/2	1 1/2	1			1/2	
38	Muesli Mix	1/2 cup (125 mL)	1 1/2				1/2	1/2	1
39	Breakfast Muesli-To-Go (2% milk choice)	1/2 recipe	2	1 1/2	2	1 1/2	1		
40	Finnish Apple Pancake (2% milk choice)	1/2 recipe	1	1 1/2	1/2	1/2	1	2	
41	Fiber-Full Bran Pancakes (2% milk choice)	1/4 recipe	1 1/2			1/2	1/2	1	
42	Individual Salsa Fresca Omelettes	1/2 recipe		1/2			2	1	
44	Overnight Broccoli and Cheese Strata (2% milk choice)	1/4 recipe	1			1	3 1/2	2	

■ Starch Foods ● Fruits & Vegetables ◆ Milk ✳ Sugars ◉ Protein Foods ▲ Fats & Oils ++ Extras

QUICK MEALS AND SNACKS — FOOD CHOICE PER SERVING

PAGE	RECIPE	SERVING SIZE	■	/	◆	✳	∅	▲	++
48	Black Bean Salsa	1/2 cup (125 mL)	1	1/2			1/2		
49	Fiery Verde Dip	1/4 cup (50 mL)	1/2				1/2		1
50	Honey-Mustard Dip (whole milk choice)	1/4 cup (50 mL)			1/2	1			
51	Quick Roasted Red Pepper Dip	1/4 cup (50 mL)		1/2			1/2	1/2	
52	Strawberry-Apple Salsa with Cinnamon Crisps	1/5 recipe	1	1/2		1		1/2	
53	No-Bake Trail Mix	1/2 cup (125 mL)	1	1				1/2	
54	Egg and Mushroom Fried Rice	1/4 recipe	2	1/2			1	1	1
55	Lunch Box Chili Rice and Beans	1	5	1/2			1		
56	Lunch Box Peachy Sweet Potato and Couscous	1	4	3 1/2					
57	Barbecued Beef Satays	1/8 recipe					2		1
58	Sticky Honey Garlic Chicken Wings	1/6 recipe				2 1/2	3	1	
59	Curried Chicken Salad Wraps	1 wrap	2	1/2			2	2	
60	Favorite Chicken Fajitas	1 fajita	2	1/2			1 1/2	1/2	
61	Hurry-Up Fill-Me-Up Burritos	1 burrito	3				1	1	
62	Swiss Chard Frittata in a Pita	1/2 recipe	2	1			3	1 1/2	
63	Tuna Salad Melt	1/8 recipe	1 1/2				1 1/2	1/2	
64	Red Pepper and Goat Cheese Pizza	1/4 recipe	2	1/2			1 1/2	2 1/2	1

SUPER SOUPS — FOOD CHOICE PER SERVING

PAGE	RECIPE	SERVING SIZE	■	/	◆	✳	∅	▲	++
68	Asian Turkey and Noodle Soup	1/6 recipe	1				2		
69	Beef, Vegetable and Bean Soup	1/8 recipe	1/2	1			2	1/2	
70	Caribbean Ham and Black Bean Soup	1/6 recipe	1 1/2	1/2			1		
71	Carrot-Orange Soup	1/6 recipe		1			1/2	1	1
72	Chilled Melon and Mango Soup	1/4 recipe		2		1			
73	Chunky Lentil and Vegetable Soup	1/6 recipe	1				1		1
74	Seafood Chowder (2% milk choice)	1/8 recipe	1/2	1/2	2		1 1/2		
75	Southwestern Sweet Potato Soup	1/6 recipe	1	1/2			1/2	1/2	1
76	Tomato and Bean Soup	1/4 recipe	1	1			1 1/2	1	

■ Starch Foods   / Fruits & Vegetables   ◆ Milk   ✳ Sugars   ∅ Protein Foods   ▲ Fats & Oils   ++ Extras

SALADS AND VEGETABLE SIDE DISHES — FOOD CHOICE PER SERVING

PAGE	RECIPE	SERVING SIZE	■	◢	◆	✳	◿	▲	++
80	Beet, Orange and Jicama Salad	1/6 recipe		1				1/2	
81	Chicken and Bean Salad	1/4 recipe	1	1/2			2 1/2		
82	Coleslaw for a Crowd	3/4 cup (175 mL)		1/2				1/2	
83	Colorful Bean and Corn Salad	1/10 recipe	1					1/2	
84	Creamy Broccoli Salad	1/6 recipe		1/2		1/2	1/2	1 1/2	
85	Cucumber Raita Salad (2% milk choice)	1/6 recipe			1/2				1
86	Fast and Easy Greek Salad	1/4 recipe		1/2			1	2	1
87	Fusilli and Fruit Salad	1/6 recipe	1	2 1/2					
88	German Potato Salad, Picnic-Style	1 cup (250 mL)	2				1/2	1/2	
89	Mandarin Orange Salad with Almonds	1/4 recipe		1		1/2	1/2	1 1/2	1
90	Penne with Asparagus and Tuna Salad	1/8 recipe	1 1/2	1/2			1 1/2		
91	Roasted Red Pepper Salad	1/6 recipe		1/2				1/2	1
92	Salmon, Potato and Green Bean Salad	1/4 recipe	1 1/2				2	1 1/2	1
93	Triple-Bean Salad with Rice and Artichokes	1/6 recipe	1 1/2	1/2			1/2	1/2	1
94	Vietnamese Rice Noodle Salad	1/6 recipe	1	1/2			2 1/2		
95	Cauliflower Casserole	1/6 recipe	1				1	1	1
96	Easy Scalloped Potatoes	1/8 recipe	1	1/2			1/2	1/2	
97	Honey Glazed Carrots	1/4 recipe		1				1/2	1
97	Sweet Potato "Fries"	1/4 recipe	1					1/2	1
98	Roasted Carrots and Parsnips	1/8 recipe		1		1/2		1	
99	Sautéed Spinach with Pine Nuts	1/4 recipe					1/2	1	1

MAIN MEALS – BEEF — FOOD CHOICE PER SERVING

PAGE	RECIPE	SERVING SIZE	■	◢	◆	✳	◿	▲	++
104	Asian Flank Steak	1/4 recipe				1 1/2	4		
105	Crockpot Beef Stew	1/4 recipe		2			3 1/2		
106	Fast Chili	1/8 recipe	1 1/2	1			3		
107	Hoisin Beef and Broccoli Stir-Fry	1/4 recipe		1/2		1/2	2 1/2		
108	Lazy Lasagna (2% milk choice)	1/8 recipe	1 1/2	1 1/2	1/2		3	1 1/2	
109	Meatloaf "Muffins" with Barbecue Sauce (2% milk choice)	1/6 recipe	1/2		1/2	1 1/2	3 1/2	2	
110	Pastitsio (2% milk choice)	1/6 recipe	1 1/2	1/2	1/2		2 1/2	1 1/2	
112	Salisbury Steak in Wine Sauce	1/6 recipe		1/2			4		1
114	Veggie, Beef and Pasta Bake	1/6 recipe	1	1			3	1 1/2	

■ Starch Foods　◢ Fruits & Vegetables　◆ Milk　✳ Sugars　◿ Protein Foods　▲ Fats & Oils　++ Extras

MAIN MEALS – PORK AND LAMB

PAGE	RECIPE	SERVING SIZE	Starch (■)	Fruits & Veg (🌿)	Milk (♦)	Sugars (✳)	Protein (⊘)	Fats & Oils (▲)	Extras (++)
115	Broiled Ham Steak with Pineapple-Mango Salsa	1/4 recipe		1 1/2			2 1/2		
116	Barbecued Butterflied Leg of Lamb	1/6 recipe					4		
117	Grilled Lamb Chops with Sautéed Peppers and Zucchini	1/4 recipe		1			2 1/2	1	
118	Polynesian Pork Kebabs	1/4 recipe		1		1/2	3 1/2		
119	Pork Chops with Peaches and Kiwi	1/4 recipe		1 1/2			3		1
120	Pork Tenderloin with Roasted Potatoes	1/3 recipe	1				4		
121	Skillet Pork Chops with Sweet Potatoes and Couscous	1/4 recipe	3	1			3 1/2		

MAIN MEALS – POULTRY

PAGE	RECIPE	SERVING SIZE	Starch (■)	Fruits & Veg (🌿)	Milk (♦)	Sugars (✳)	Protein (⊘)	Fats & Oils (▲)	Extras (++)
122	Baked Chicken and Potato Dinner	1/4 recipe	2				4 1/2		
123	Baked Chicken Parmesan	1/4 recipe		1			6 1/2		
124	Chinese Almond Chicken with Noodles	1/4 recipe	3	1/2			4		
126	Creamy Bow-Ties with Chicken, Spinach and Peppers (2% milk choice)	1/4 recipe	2	1/2	1		4	1/2	
128	Creole Crockpot Chicken	1/8 recipe		1			4	1/2	
129	Curried Chicken with Apples and Bananas (2% milk choice)	1/6 recipe		1 1/2	1/2		3 1/2		
130	Curried Red Pepper Chicken	1/6 recipe		1/2			3		
131	Hot 'n' Spicy Turkey Burgers	1/4 recipe	2 1/2			1/2	3	1	
132	Skillet Chicken and Shrimp Paella	1/6 recipe	2	1			3		
134	Turkey Pot Pie with Biscuit Topping (2% milk choice)	1/6 recipe	1 1/2	1 1/2	1/2		3 1/2	1/2	
136	Exotic Ginger-Cumin Chicken	1/8 recipe		1			4		

MAIN MEALS – FISH

PAGE	RECIPE	SERVING SIZE	Starch (■)	Fruits & Veg (🌿)	Milk (♦)	Sugars (✳)	Protein (⊘)	Fats & Oils (▲)	Extras (++)
137	Crunchy Fish Burgers	1/4 recipe	4	1/2		1/2	3 1/2		
138	Parmesan-Herb Baked Fish Fillets	1/4 recipe	1/2	1/2			3		
139	Pasta with White Clam Sauce (2% milk choice)	1/4 recipe	3	1/2	1/2		3		
140	Quick Steamed Fish Fillets with Potatoes and Asparagus	1/2 recipe	1				3		
141	Salmon with Roasted Vegetables	1/2 recipe	1	1 1/2			3	2	
142	Shrimp and Mussels with Couscous	1/4 recipe	3 1/2	1			1 1/2		
143	Spaghettini with Tuna, Olives and Capers	1/4 recipe	2 1/2	1 1/2			2	1/2	1
144	Tuna and Rice Casserole (2% milk choice)	1/4 recipe	1 1/2	1/2	1/2		2	1	1

■ Starch Foods 🌿 Fruits & Vegetables ♦ Milk ✳ Sugars ⊘ Protein Foods ▲ Fats & Oils ++ Extras

Main Meals – Pasta and Legumes

FOOD CHOICE PER SERVING

PAGE	RECIPE	SERVING SIZE	■	🍃	◆	✳	◙	▲	✛✛
145	Chickpea Hot Pot	1/6 recipe	1	1 1/2			1 1/2		
146	Creamy Pasta and Broccoli	1/6 recipe	3				1	1 1/2	
147	Crowd Pleasing Vegetarian Chili	1/6 recipe	3 1/2	1/2			1	1	
148	Fettuccine Carbonara	1/4 recipe	4	1/2			3	1	
149	Pasta with Roasted Vegetables and Goat Cheese	1/4 recipe	2 1/2	1			1	2	1
150	Piquant Tomato Sauce	1/8 recipe		1 1/2				1	
151	Penne with Mushrooms and Spicy Tomato Sauce	1/4 recipe	2 1/2	1 1/2			1	1 1/2	
152	Rotini with Vegetable Tomato Sauce	1/4 recipe	2 1/2	2			1	1	
153	Spinach and Mushroom Pizza Pie	1/6 recipe	3 1/2	1/2			1 1/2	3	
154	Teriyaki Tofu Stir-Fry	1/4 recipe	2	1		1/2	1	1/2	

Fast Finishes

FOOD CHOICE PER SERVING

PAGE	RECIPE	SERVING SIZE	■	🍃	◆	✳	◙	▲	✛✛
158	Apricot Bread Pudding (2% milk choice)	1/8 recipe	1	1	1/2	2 1/2	1/2	1	
159	Awesome Pineapple Cake	1/12 recipe	1	1		3 1/2		2 1/2	
160	Cranberry Oatmeal Cookies	2 cookies	1			1/2		1	
161	Cold Maple Mousse	1/10 recipe				2		3 1/2	
162	Country Apple Berry Crisp	1/4 recipe	1	2 1/2		2 1/2		2 1/2	
163	Date and Oatmeal Cake with Mocha Frosting	1/16 recipe	1/2	1		2		2	
164	Fresh Strawberry Pie	1/6 recipe	1	1/2		1		1 1/2	
165	Lunchbox Applesauce Cake	1/9 recipe	1 1/2			2 1/2		2	
166	Luscious Lemon Bars	1 large bar	1/2			1 1/2		1 1/2	
168	Orange Crème Caramel (2% milk choice)	1/8 recipe			1/2	2 1/2	1/2	1/2	
169	Peach Cobbler	1/6 recipe	1	1/2		1		1/2	
170	Pear Gingerbread Upside-Down Cake	1/12 recipe	1	1		2		1 1/2	

■ Starch Foods   🍃 Fruits & Vegetables   ◆ Milk   ✳ Sugars   ◙ Protein Foods   ▲ Fats & Oils   ✛✛ Extras

INDEX